Case-Based Simulation and Review for USMLE Step 2 CS

Case-Based Simulation and Review for USMLE Step 2 CS

Theodore X. O'Connell, MD

Associate Program Director and
Director of Residency Research Curriculum
Family Medicine Residency Program
Kaiser Permanente Woodland Hills
Woodland Hills, California
Clinical Instructor
Department of Family Medicine
David Geffen School of Medicine at UCLA
Los Angeles, California
Partner Physician
Southern California Permanente Medical Group
Woodland Hills, California

Timothy J. Horita, MD

Program Director
Family Medicine Residency Program
Kaiser Permanente Woodland Hills
Woodland Hills, California
Clinical Assistant Professor
Department of Family Medicine
David Geffen School of Medicine at UCLA
Los Angeles, California
Partner Physician
Southern California Permanente Medical Group
Woodland Hills, California

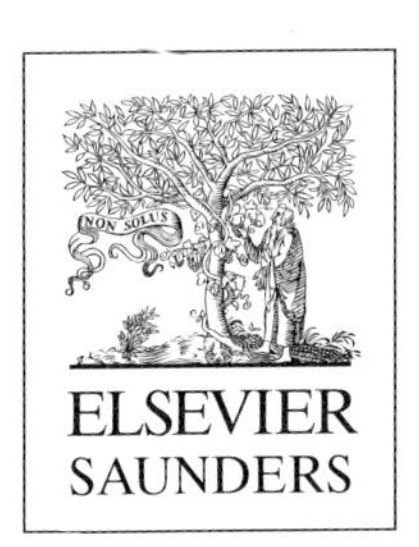

ELSEVIER
SAUNDERS

ELSEVIER
SAUNDERS

1600 John F. Kennedy Boulevard
Suite 1800
Philadelphia, PA 19103-2899

CASE-BASED SIMULATION AND REVIEW FOR USMLE STEP 2 CS ISBN 13: 978-1-4160-2547-4
ISBN 10: 1-4160-2547-2

Notice

Knowledge and best practice in this field are constantly changing. As new research and experience broaden our knowledge, changes in practice, treatment and drug therapy may become necessary or appropriate. Readers are advised to check the most current information provided (i) on procedures featured or (ii) by the manufacturer of each product to be administered, to verify the recommended dose or formula, the method and duration of administration, and contraindications. It is the responsibility of the practitioner, relying on his or her own experience and knowledge of the patient, to make diagnoses, to determine dosages and the best treatment for each individual patient, and to take all appropriate safety precautions. To the fullest extent of the law, neither the Publisher nor the Editor assumes any liability for any injury and/or damage to persons or property arising out or related to any use of the material contained in this book.

International Standard Book Number: 1-4160-2547-2

Acquisitions Editor: Jim Merritt
Editorial Assistant: Nicole DiCicco
Senior Project Manager: Cecelia Bayruns
Marketing Manager: Kate Rubin

Printed in the United States of America.

Last digit is the print number: 9 8 7 6 5 4 3 2 1

To my wife, Nichole, for her constant love and support,
and to my tenth grade English teacher, Mr. Terry Caldwell,
for teaching me to write.

Ted O'Connell

To my wife, Andrea, for allowing me the time to pursue
my academic and professional ambitions.
To my sons, Henry, Josh, and Jacob, do your homework!

Tim Horita

About the Authors

Theodore X. O'Connell, M.D., is the associate program director of the Kaiser Permanente Woodland Hills Family Medicine Residency Program where he also directs the residency research curriculum. Dr. O'Connell is a partner in the Southern California Permanente Medical Group and is a clinical instructor in the Department of Family Medicine at the David Geffen School of Medicine at UCLA. He is the recipient of numerous clinical, teaching, and research awards. Dr. O'Connell has been published widely as the author of textbook chapters, review books, journal articles, and editorials. He received his medical degree from the University of California, Los Angeles School of Medicine and completed a residency and chief residency at Santa Monica-UCLA Medical Center in Santa Monica, California.

Timothy J. Horita, M.D., is the program director of the Kaiser Permanente Woodland Hills Family Medicine Residency Program. Dr. Horita is a partner in the Southern California Permanente Medical Group and is a clinical assistant professor in the Department of Family Medicine at the David Geffen School of Medicine at UCLA. He has been the recipient of several teaching awards. Dr. Horita received his medical degree from Dartmouth Medical School and completed a residency and chief residency at Kaiser Permanente Medical Center in Woodland Hills, California.

Contents

About the USMLE Step 2 CS

The USMLE Step 2 Clinical Skills (CS) examination is a pass/fail examination designed to mirror a physician's typical workday in various clinical settings. This is a 1-day test in which examinees will interview and examine 11 or 12 standardized patients. The standardized patients are individuals trained to portray real patients and test one's clinical skills. The cases will cover common and important situations that a physician is likely to encounter in medical practice in clinics, doctor's offices, emergency departments, and hospital settings in the United States.

The purpose of the Step 2 CS is to assess whether an examinee can demonstrate the fundamental clinical skills essential to safe and effective patient care under supervision. The clinical skills being tested include taking a relevant medical history, performing an appropriate physical examination, communicating effectively with the patient, clearly and accurately documenting the findings and diagnostic hypotheses from the clinical encounter, and ordering appropriate initial diagnostic studies.

Examinees will be given approximately 15 minutes for each encounter. During the encounter they are expected to establish rapport with the standardized patient, elicit pertinent historical information, perform a focused physical examination, communicate effectively, and clearly document findings and diagnostic impressions. Most cases are designed to elicit a process of history taking and physical examination that demonstrates the examinee's ability to list and pursue various possible diagnoses. Some cases, however, may focus only on history taking or on physical examination.

After each patient encounter, the examinee will be given additional time to record a progress note reflecting the encounter. This note can be handwritten or entered into a custom-designed software program on computers that will be available. The progress note should include pertinent history and physical examination findings, diagnostic impressions, and plans for further evaluation if necessary.

The intent of this examination is to ensure that examinees encounter a broad spectrum of cases reflecting common and important symptoms and diagnoses. Topics include cardiovascular, gastrointestinal, genitourinary, musculoskeletal, neurological, psychiatric, respiratory, constitutional, and women's health. The selection of cases is also guided by specifications relating to acuity, age, gender, and type of physical findings presented in each case.

Examinees are scored in three separate components: Integrated Clinical Encounter (ICE), Communication and Interpersonal Skills (CIS), and Spoken English Proficiency (SEP). Each of these individual components must be passed in order to achieve a passing performance on Step 2 CS.

Integrated Clinical Encounter (ICE)

The ICE assesses one's ability to gather data and document it appropriately. Data gathering consists of patient information collected by history taking and physical examination. Documentation is assessed through the completion of a patient note summarizing the findings of the patient encounter as well as the diagnostic impression and the initial patient workup.

Data gathering is scored by checklists that are completed by the standardized patients. These checklists are developed by committees of clinicians and medical school clinical faculty, and are intended to comprise the essential history and physical examination elements for specific clinical encounters. The patient note is scored by trained physician raters. Copies of the patient note template, sample patient note styles, and software to practice typing the note are available on the USMLE Web site at *www.usmle.org*.

Communication and Interpersonal Skills (CIS)

The CIS includes an assessment of questioning skills, information sharing skills, and professional manner and rapport. The questioning skills focus on the use of open-ended questions, transitional statements, and how to allow the patient to speak without being interrupted. Information sharing skills determine whether the examinee avoids the use of jargon, responds well to patient questions and concerns, and provides counseling when appropriate. Professional manner and rapport assesses the examinee's concern for the patient's comfort and modesty, as well as the examinee's attention to personal hygiene. It also focuses on whether the examinee expresses interest in the impact of the illness on the patient.

Spoken English Proficiency (SEP)

The SEP includes an assessment of clarity of spoken English communication within the context of the doctor-patient encounter. Specifically, items such as pronunciation, word choice, and minimizing the need to repeat questions or statements are assessed.

SEP performance is assessed by the standardized patients using rating scales and is based upon the frequency of pronunciation or word choice errors that affect comprehension. In addition, the amount of listener effort required to understand the examinee's questions and responses is assessed.

Why You Need This Book!

Why You Need This Book!

The mere thought of the USMLE Step 2 CS is anxiety-provoking for many medical students. Not only are your clinical skills and knowledge on display, but you also have a significant financial investment on the line. This book will help you prepare for this exam in the most helpful way possible: by simulating the clinical scenarios similar to those you might experience during the real exam. In addition to providing the appropriate clinical scenarios, this book provides case-based discussions on the topics likely to be encountered during the Step 2 CS.

This book is designed to serve two purposes. First, the cases presented reflect symptoms and diagnoses that will mirror what you will see on the Step 2 CS examination. The cases presented in this book will serve you best if you use them as case studies, preferably in a group format with your classmates. By treating each case as a real-life interaction and a representation of the Step 2 CS, you will gain confidence with the format of the test. Not only must you interact with the patient, but you also will become more comfortable with this type of observational setting. In essence, practice makes perfect, and properly utilizing these cases will improve your performance on the real examination.

Second, the information following each case should serve as a study guide focusing on the important elements of the history and physical examination of each case. The clinical data provided reflects the most up-to-date recommendations from national organizations such as the American Diabetes Association, the American Thoracic Society, the International Headache Society, and JNC 7.

By using this book in the intended manner, you should find yourself comfortable going into the actual examination, both with the setting and with the clinical topics.

Specifics Regarding the Examination

Items to Bring to the Examination

You should bring the following items to the examination:

- An acceptable form of government-issued identification.
- A clean, white laboratory or clinic coat. Your name and institution will be covered with adhesive tape by the proctors.
- A stethoscope.

No other medical equipment is necessary and will not be allowed into the examination. All necessary equipment will be provided in the examination rooms.

Attire

It is recommended that you wear comfortable professional clothing to the examination. Though this is open to interpretation, we recommend that you err on the side of more conservative attire since you will be scored on professional appearance and attitude, which is a subjective measure.

Items Not Allowed at the Examination

The following items are not allowed at the examination and may not be used during breaks in the exam:

- Cellular telephones
- Pagers
- Two-way communication devices
- Personal digital assistants (PDAs)
- Digital watches

Examination Length

The entire examination lasts approximately 8 hours, interrupted by two breaks. You will be served a light meal during the first break and may bring your own food as long as refrigeration and preparation are not required. Smoking is prohibited in the examination centers.

The examination will consist of 11 or 12 patient encounters. A few of the patient encounters may be used to pilot test new cases and will not be used in determining your score on the examination.

Equipment

The testing area consists of a series of examination rooms that are equipped with sinks, paper towels, and examination tables. Appropriate diagnostic equipment such as blood pressure cuffs, examination gloves, otoscopes, ophthalmoscopes, and reflex hammers will be provided.

The Patient Encounter

Before each patient encounter, examinee instructions will be posted on the examination room door for your review. The examinee instructions provide specific instructions, as well as basic patient information and the reason for the visit. Vital signs are provided and should be accepted as accurate (you do not need to measure them again).

Upon entering the examination room, you will encounter the standardized patient. Introduce yourself as "student doctor (your name)" and offer to shake the patient's hand. Ask the patient his or her chief complaint, or confirm the chief complaint that was provided on the instruction sheet. You should then ask historical questions relevant to the patient's chief complaint. You do not need to perform a complete history and physical exam on each patient. The questions you ask should be relevant to the case. Remember to obtain information such as social history and family history when it seems relevant.

After you have obtained the appropriate historical information, perform an appropriate physical examination. Do not forget to wash your hands prior to examining the patient. Perform the examination as you would on any patient with the same presenting complaint. However, certain parts of the physical exam should not be performed. These include genitourinary, rectal, pelvic, female breast, and invasive ocular examinations (such as the corneal reflex). If you would normally perform one of the parts of the physical exam for a certain complaint, you should include it as part of your proposed diagnostic evaluation. You may also state to the standardized patient that you would perform that part of the exam, and the standardized patient may provide you with the findings of the examination.

During the physical examination, you should perform all maneuvers correctly, as you would with a real patient. There may be positive physical findings present, some of which will be simulated by the patient. Alternatively, you may be told the abnormal findings of certain parts of the examination by the standardized patient as you perform them. Any of these findings, positive or negative, should be considered in determining your differential diagnosis.

After obtaining an appropriate history and performing a focused physical examination, you should be able to develop a preliminary differential diagnosis and a plan for a diagnostic evaluation. The exam will assess whether you communicate with the standardized patients in a professional and empathetic manner. As you would when encountering real patients, you should answer any questions they may have. In addition, you should tell them what diagnoses you are considering, as well as what tests and studies you plan to order to clarify their diagnoses.

In each case, you will be given approximately 15 minutes to complete the patient encounter. You will be instructed when to begin the patient encounter, and will hear an announcement when there are 5 minutes remaining. Another announcement will be made indicating that the patient encounter is over. If you complete the patient encounter in fewer than 15 minutes, you may leave the examination room early, but you will not be allowed to re-enter.

The Progress Note

After the encounter with the patient, you will have 10 minutes to complete a progress note. If you finish with the encounter before the allotted 15 minutes have passed, you may also use this time to complete your note.

The progress note should be the same type of note that you would write for a typical patient encounter. The note should be thorough yet concise. The pertinent medical history, findings of the physical examination (including vital signs), and any available laboratory data or diagnostic studies should be included. The note should also include your working differential diagnosis, as well as a treatment plan. The treatment plan should include any diagnostic studies that you think are appropriate, as well as the parts of the exam that are indicated but are not performed (rectal, pelvic, female breast exam, etc.). *Specific treatments, consultations, or referrals should not be included in the treatment plan.* If you think that no diagnostic workup is indicated for a particular case, write "no studies indicated" rather than leaving the treatment plan section blank.

The patient note may be handwritten or entered on a computer that will be available. If you have poor handwriting, we recommend that you use the computer to type the progress note, since illegible handwriting may adversely affect your score if the graders are not able to identify what you are writing. If you are going to hand write the progress note, do not touch the computer keyboard, as it will create a blank progress note.

The USMLE Web site, located at *www.usmle.org*, provides sample patient notes, as well as a blank patient note screen similar to what will appear on the computers that will be provided. We suggest that you visit the Web site to familiarize yourself with these samples to become more comfortable with the expected format.

Using This Book

Each case in this book is presented in approximately the same format. We suggest that one student act as the standardized patient, one student score the interaction based upon the checklist provided and the written progress note, and one student take the test as the examinee. In doing so, each student will be exposed to a different aspect of the case and can learn from it in that manner.

You may learn from other students' interview styles, as well as the questions they pose to the patient and their examination techniques. You may even consider repeating the case while playing different roles to improve your performance on the examination.

After the case has been completed, use the study guide as a group to review the important aspects of the history and physical exam that should have been completed. Then review the current clinical recommendations, which also are provided.

The format of each case is presented as follows:

- *The examinee prompt.* This should be read by the examinee prior to entering the examination room.
- *The standardized patient information.* The student playing the standardized patient should commit as much of this information to memory as possible. The information is presented in the usual format of a thorough history and physical exam. Be sure to understand the pertinent positives in the physical exam, and be prepared to act them out. In some cases, vital signs are provided. The page on which the vital signs are provided will indicate when you should provide them to the examiner. Finally, pertinent laboratory or x-ray data is presented for some of the cases and should be made available to the examiner if requested. Specific instructions are provided with each case.
- *Data gathering scoring checklist.* This checklist can be scored either by the student acting as the standardized patient, or by another student who is responsible only for scoring the interaction. We recommend that the case be scored by someone other than the standardized patient so that the standardized patient can better stay in character and interact effectively with the examinee. The scoring of each case is based upon subjective, objective, assessment, and plan components of the interaction. Details regarding scoring each case are provided in the next chapter.
- *Study guide.* At the end of each case study, a study guide is provided that outlines current diagnostic and therapeutic recommendations regarding the case at hand. This study guide may be used either for group or individual study, but the essentials provided should be well-understood prior to taking the real Step 2 CS.

Scoring the Clinical Scenario

Scoring each case is based upon both subjective as well as objective data. Checklists are provided to guide the scoring, but may be subject to interpretation. During the actual USMLE Step 2, data gathering is scored by checklists that are completed by the standardized patients. The patient note is scored by trained physician raters. Obviously, this leaves some aspects of the examination open to clinical judgment. Likewise, during these practice clinical scenarios, the students doing the scoring may need to apply judgment to provide a score.

The following information outlines the scoring for each case:

- The subjective portion evaluates whether the examinee has asked the appropriate questions relative to the case. The objective portion evaluates the physical exam, which should be problem-focused yet thorough. The scoring of the assessment and plan is based upon the written portion of the progress note that is completed by the examiner after the interview and examination with the standardized patient. Scoring scales are provided that will evaluate competency regarding the case.

  The standardized patient should complete the subjective and objective portions of the checklist on the scoring sheet. Another student can then use the checklist to score the progress note. The subjective and objective portions of the scoring sheet should also be completed by the student scoring the progress note, because some of the items, such as vital signs or a general assessment of the patient, may appear in the progress note but may not necessarily be spoken to the standardized patient.

  Finally, once the scoring sheet is completed, add up the number of boxes that were checked as being appropriate and correct. A score of 70% of the total points possible is considered a passing score in this book, although scoring by the USMLE may differ. The number needed for a "passing" score is included with each case.
- *Communication and Interpersonal Skills rating scale*. Each case comes with a second scoring sheet that is used to evaluate the communication and interpersonal skills of the examinee. As with the other scoring sheet, this may be completed either by the standardized patient or an independent evaluator. A score of 70% of the total points possible is considered a passing score in this book, although scoring by the USMLE may differ. This "passing" score is provided on each scoring sheet.

  You may find it difficult to grade a fellow classmate on communication style, but an honest evaluation can be used to provide constructive feedback, and ultimately may result in a higher score on the actual examination.
- *Spoken English Proficiency rating scale*. Each case comes with a third scoring sheet that is used to evaluate the examinee's proficiency with the English language. It focuses on pronunciation, word choice, and clarity in speaking with the patient. This scoresheet may be completed either by the standardized patient or an independent evaluator. A score of 70% of the total points possible is considered a passing score in this book, although scoring by the USMLE may differ. This "passing" score is provided on each scoring sheet. Again, you may find it difficult to critique a classmate, but honest feedback can be beneficial.

"I'm Here about My Sugars"

Examinee Prompt

You have inherited a patient who was previously treated by Dr. Smith. The patient is a 47-year-old man with type II diabetes who has not been to see a doctor in over 1 year. Your nurse reports that the patient is here today to follow up on his diabetes. Attached you will find the patient's lab work from his last doctor's visit. Please perform the following procedures:

- ❑ Obtain a focused history relevant to this patient's medical status.
- ❑ Conduct an appropriate physical examination.

You have 15 minutes for your interaction with the patient. Following your visit with the patient, you will be asked to write a progress note regarding the visit. Please include the pertinent aspects of the visit in the subjective and objective portions of the note. Please include an assessment as well as a treatment plan, which should include your treatment goals for this patient's HbA1C, low-density lipoprotein (LDL) cholesterol, and blood pressure. You have an additional 10 minutes to complete the progress note following your encounter with the patient.

Lab Work for This Patient

Fasting blood glucose	197
HbA1C	7.6
Total cholesterol	242
High-density lipoprotein (HDL)	52
LDL	134
Triglycerides	185

Vital Signs

Blood pressure	152/92 mm Hg
Heart rate	70
Respiratory rate	14
Height	70 inches
Weight	230 pounds

Patient Prompt

Background: You are a 47-year-old patient who was diagnosed with type II diabetes 5 years ago. You used to see Dr. Smith on a regular basis; however, you have been busy with work and have not been able to get in to see the doctor in over 1 year. You are transferring your care to this new doctor.

Chief Complaint: Diabetes follow-up

History of the Present Illness: 47-year-old man here for follow-up of diabetes. Has not had any medical care in over 1 year. No specific complaints.

Past Medical History:

- Type II diabetes mellitus diagnosed 5 years ago
- No acute or chronic complications
- Last ophthalmologic exam 2 years ago
- Hypertension

Past Surgical History: None

Medications: Metformin 500 mg bid. You have always been on this treatment regimen. You do not take any vitamins or nutritional supplements.

Allergies: No known drug allergies

Family History: Father had a history of diabetes and died of a heart attack at age 58. Mother is alive and healthy.

Social History:

- Works as a retail sales manager
- Married, 2 children
- Smokes 1/2 pack cigarettes per day for the last 20 years
- Two alcoholic drinks per week
- No drug use
- Exercises only rarely
- Diet is "fair"

Review of Systems: Negative

Additional Information:

- You check your blood glucose about once per week, and it runs from 160 to 200.
- The physical exam findings are normal.

Scoring

Subjective

- ❑ Duration of diabetes diagnosis
- ❑ Past medical history
- ❑ Medications
- ❑ Family history
- ❑ Smoking history
- ❑ Dietary habits
- ❑ Exercise habits

Objective

- ❑ Blood pressure
- ❑ Funduscopic exam
- ❑ Cardiovascular exam
- ❑ Pulmonary exam
- ❑ Foot exam (must include monofilament exam)

Assessment

- ❑ Type II diabetes, not adequately controlled
- ❑ Hypertension
- ❑ Hyperlipidemia
- ❑ Tobacco use
- ❑ Obesity

Plan (credit for up to five of the following items)

- ❑ Aspirin therapy
- ❑ A retinal photograph or ophthalmologic exam
- ❑ Smoking cessation program or advise patient to quit smoking
- ❑ A diet and exercise program with follow-up of HbA1C or appropriate change in diabetes medication
- ❑ A diet and exercise program with follow-up of blood pressure or implementing blood pressure medication
- ❑ A diet and exercise program with follow-up lipid panel or implementing cholesterol lowering medication (statin)
- ❑ Measurement of microalbumin
- ❑ Measurement of serum creatinine

Total Score: ____ / 22

Passing score for this station is 15 correct items.

Communication And Interpersonal Skills (CIS) Scoresheet

Please rate each of the following items on a scale from 1–10.
These items may be completed by either the standardized patient or another student.

Scoresheet 1

	Poor		Fair		Good		Very Good		Excellent	
Professional appearance	1	2	3	4	5	6	7	8	9	10
Introduces self and shakes hands	1	2	3	4	5	6	7	8	9	10
Nonverbal communication (eye contact, facial expressiveness, body language)	1	2	3	4	5	6	7	8	9	10
Communicates effectively (open-ended questions, avoids jargon)	1	2	3	4	5	6	7	8	9	10
Establishes rapport with patient (empathy, appears nonjudgmental)	1	2	3	4	5	6	7	8	9	10
Allows patient to speak without being interrupted	1	2	3	4	5	6	7	8	9	10
Listens and seems to understand patient's concerns	1	2	3	4	5	6	7	8	9	10
Overall professionalism	1	2	3	4	5	6	7	8	9	10

Total Score:

Passing score for CIS section is 56 points.

Spoken English Proficiency (SEP) Scoresheet

Please rate each of the following items on a scale from 1–10.
These items may be completed by either the standardized patient or another student.

Scoresheet 2

	Poor		Fair		Good		Very Good		Excellent	
Examiner is articulate and easily understood	1	2	3	4	5	6	7	8	9	10
Pronunciation (words pronounced correctly; accent does not hinder communication)	1	2	3	4	5	6	7	8	9	10
Word choice is appropriate	1	2	3	4	5	6	7	8	9	10
Ability to communicate without excessive listener effort required to understand questions or responses	1	2	3	4	5	6	7	8	9	10
Patient's ability to understand the examiner	1	2	3	4	5	6	7	8	9	10
Examiner's ability to understand the patient	1	2	3	4	5	6	7	8	9	10

Total Score:

Passing score for SEP section is 42 points.

Standards of Medical Care in Type II Diabetes Mellitus

Diagnosis

Diabetes mellitus may be diagnosed in three ways:

1. Fasting plasma glucose of 126 mg/dL (the preferred test)
2. Symptoms of diabetes (polyuria, polydipsia, and unexplained weight loss) and casual plasma glucose of 200 mg/dL
3. Two-hour postprandial glucose of 200 mg/dL during a 75-g oral glucose tolerance test

Medical History

The following items should be included in the medical history:

1. Symptoms, results of laboratory tests, and special examination results related to the diagnosis of diabetes
2. Prior HbA1C records
3. Eating patterns, nutritional status, and weight history
4. Details of previous treatment programs, including nutrition and diabetes self-management education, attitudes, and health beliefs
5. Current treatment of diabetes, including medications, meal plan, and results of glucose monitoring
6. Exercise history
7. History of acute complications such as ketoacidosis and hypoglycemia
8. Prior or current infections, particularly skin, foot, dental, and genitourinary infections
9. Symptoms and treatment of chronic complications associated with diabetes (such as eye, kidney, nerve, genitourinary, bladder, gastrointestinal function, heart, peripheral vascular, foot, and cerebrovascular)
10. Other medications that may affect blood glucose levels
11. Risk factors for atherosclerosis: smoking, hypertension, obesity, dyslipidemia, and family history
12. History and treatment of other conditions
13. Family history
14. Lifestyle, cultural, psychosocial, educational, and economic factors that might influence the management of diabetes
15. Tobacco, alcohol, and/or controlled substance use

Physical Examination

1. Height and weight
2. Blood pressure determination
3. Funduscopic examination
4. Oral examination
5. Thyroid palpation
6. Cardiac examination
7. Abdominal examination (e.g., for hepatomegaly)
8. Evaluation of pulses by palpation and with auscultation
9. Hand/finger examination
10. Foot examination, including a monofilament exam
11. Skin examination (for acanthosis nigricans and insulin-injection sites)
12. Neurologic examination

Comprehensive Laboratory Evaluation

1. HbA1C
2. Fasting lipid profile, including total cholesterol, HDL cholesterol, triglycerides, and LDL cholesterol
3. Test for microalbuminuria
4. Serum creatinine in adults
5. Thyroid-stimulating hormone (TSH) in all type I diabetic patients; in type II if clinically indicated
6. Liver function tests for those on statin medications
7. Electrocardiogram in adults, if clinically indicated
8. Urinalysis for ketones, protein, sediment

Management Recommendations

Glycemic Control

1. HbA1C goal is <7.0%. Perform this test at least two times per year in patients who are meeting treatment goals and quarterly in patients whose therapy has changed or who are not meeting glycemic goals.
2. Self-monitoring of blood glucose (SMBG) is an integral component of diabetes therapy.

3. A regular physical activity program is recommended for all patients with diabetes who are able to participate.

Blood Pressure

1. Blood pressure should be measured at every routine diabetes visit. Goal blood pressure is <130/80 mm Hg.
2. Patients with a systolic blood pressure of 130 to 139 mm Hg or a diastolic blood pressure of 80 to 90 mm Hg should be given lifestyle and behavioral therapy alone for a maximum of 3 months.
3. Initial drug therapy for those with a blood pressure >140/90 mm Hg should be treated with a drug class shown to reduce cardiovascular events in patients with diabetes [angiotensin-converting enzyme inhibitors (ACE), angiotensin-receptor blockers (ARB), β-blockers, diuretics, and calcium channel blockers].
4. All patients with diabetes and hypertension should be treated with a regimen that includes either an ACE inhibitor or an ARB. These medications require monitoring of renal function and serum potassium levels.

Lipid Management

1. Test for lipid disorders at least annually and more often if needed to achieve goals. Goal lipid values are LDL <100 mg/dL, triglycerides <150 mg/dL, and HDL 1.40 mg/dL.
2. Lifestyle modification focusing on the reduction of saturated fat and cholesterol intake, weight loss, increased physical activity, and smoking cessation has been shown to improve the lipid profile in patients with diabetes.
3. Patients who do not achieve lipid goals with lifestyle modifications require pharmacologic therapy. Statin medications have been shown to be associated with a reduction in cardiovascular events.

Aspirin Therapy

1. Use aspirin therapy as a secondary prevention strategy in those with diabetes with a history of myocardial infarction, vascular bypass procedure, stroke or transient ischemic attack, peripheral vascular disease, claudication, and/or angina.
2. Use aspirin therapy as a primary prevention strategy in those who are over 40 years of age or who have additional risk factors (hypertension, smoking, dyslipidemia, albuminuria, or family history of cardiovascular disease).

Smoking Cessation

1. Advise all patients not to smoke.
2. Include smoking cessation counseling and other forms of treatment as a routine component of diabetes care.

Cardiovascular Disease Screening

1. Candidates for a screening cardiac stress test include the following groups. (However, it should be noted that there is no current evidence that such testing in asymptomatic patients with risk factors improves outcomes).
   - Those with a history of peripheral or carotid vascular disease.
   - Those with a sedentary lifestyle who are over age 35, and plan to begin a vigorous exercise regimen.
   - Those with two or more cardiac risk factors.
2. In patients with treated congestive heart failure, metformin use is contraindicated.
3. In patients >55 years of age, with or without hypertension but with another cardiovascular risk factor, an ACE inhibitor should be considered to reduce the risk of cardiovascular events.
4. In patients with a prior myocardial infarction or in patients undergoing major surgery, β-blockers should be considered in addition to an ACE inhibitor to reduce mortality.

Nephropathy Screening and Treatment

1. Perform an annual test for the presence of microalbuminuria.
2. In the treatment of both micro- and macroalbuminuria, either ACE inhibitors or ARBs should be used.
3. With the presence of nephropathy, initiate protein restriction to <0.8 g/kg of body weight per day.

Diabetic Retinopathy

1. Patients with type II diabetes should have an annual dilated eye examination by an ophthalmologist or optometrist who is experienced in diagnosing the presence of

diabetic retinopathy and is aware of its management.

Foot Care

1. Perform a comprehensive foot examination annually on patients with diabetes. Perform a visual inspection of patient's feet at each routine visit.
2. The foot examination should include the use of a Semmes-Weinstein monofilament, tuning fork, palpation, and visual examination.
3. Refer high-risk patients to foot care specialists for ongoing preventive care.
4. Refer patients with significant claudication or a positive ankle-brachial index for further vascular assessment.

Vaccinations

1. Annually provide an influenza vaccine to all diabetic patients 6 months of age or older.
2. Provide at least one lifetime pneumococcal vaccine for adults with diabetes.

REFERENCES

American Diabetes Association. Standards of medical care in diabetes. Diabetes Care 2004;27:S15–S35.

"I Think I Have a Brain Tumor"

Examinee Prompt

You are seeing this 38-year-old woman, who is a new patient to you, for a chief complaint of "headache." Please complete the following tasks:

- ❑ Obtain a focused history relevant to the patient's chief complaint.
- ❑ Perform an appropriate focused physical exam.

You have 15 minutes for your visit with this patient. Please discuss your diagnosis and plan with the patient model at this station. When you have all of the information and have completed your discussion with the patient, you may leave the exam room. Following the patient encounter, please write a progress note in standard "SOAP" (Subjective, Objective, Assessment and Plan) format. You will have 10 additional minutes to complete your progress note.

Vital Signs

Temperature . . . . 98.6°F
Blood pressure . . . . 128/74 mm Hg
Pulse 74
Respiratory rate 15

Patient Prompt

Background: You are a 38-year-old patient complaining of headaches for the last 20 years. You have been told by friends and family that you have "migraines" and you are convinced that these headaches are in fact migraines after researching the topic on the Internet.

Chief Complaint: Headaches

History of the Present Illness: 38-year-old woman with a long-standing history of mild to moderate (3 to 6 out of 10 in intensity) bitemporal or occipital headaches. You describe them as a pressure-like sensation with gradual onset. You deny any throbbing sensation. They occur two to four times per month without significant change in their pattern. You have not missed work or social functions due to these headaches. You usually take nothing but occasionally take over-the-counter medications such as ibuprofen or Excedrin with good results. The headaches improve somewhat with physical activity.

Past Medical and Surgical History: None

Medications: Ibuprofen 400 to 600 mg daily; Excedrin 2 to 3 tablets daily

Allergies: No known drug allergies

Family History: Noncontributory

Social History: Married for 10 years
No children
Work part-time as an accountant
You deny any tobacco, alcohol, or drug use
You don't regularly exercise

Review of Systems: No history of head trauma. No nausea or vomiting. Occasionally you have mild light sensitivity but this is rare. No phonophobia. No fevers. No weakness, numbness, paresthesias, or dizziness. No preceding aura. No visual disturbance or scotomata. You deny any changes in mental status, confusion, or difficulty with speech.

Additional Information:

- You have a neighbor who had a brain tumor and you are worried that your headaches may be a sign of this.
- You are convinced at first that you need an MRI (magnetic resonance imaging) of your brain "just to be sure." Be fairly insistent on this at first. After 10 minutes, if the examinee provides an adequate level of reassurance, you can abandon this issue.
- All physical exam findings are normal.

Scoring Sheet for Headache Station

Subjective

- ❑ Asks chief complaint
- ❑ Location of pain
- ❑ Frequency
- ❑ Severity
- ❑ Aggravating/alleviating factors
- ❑ Nausea/vomiting
- ❑ Light/sound sensitivity
- ❑ Fevers
- ❑ Neurologic symptoms (credit for any of the following: numbness, weakness, difficulty with speech, mental status problems, visual changes)
- ❑ Frequency of symptoms
- ❑ Medications
- ❑ Past medical history
- ❑ History of trauma
- ❑ Social history (credit for any of the following: job, marital status, smoking, alcohol)

Objective

- ❑ Funduscopic exam
- ❑ Cranial nerves II through XII examined
- ❑ Palpation of scalp and neck for focal tenderness or reproduction of symptoms
- ❑ Evaluation for meningismus/neck stiffness
- ❑ Evaluation for gross sensory deficits
- ❑ Evaluation for gross motor deficits
- ❑ Assessment of gait

Diagnosis (other items in the differential diagnosis on the progress note do not need to be scored)

- ❑ Correct diagnosis of tension-type headache

Plan

- ❑ Plan does not include neuroimaging
- ❑ Indicates a follow-up plan

Total Score: _____ / 24

Passing score for this station is 17 correct items.

Communication and Interpersonal Skills (CIS) Scoresheet

Please rate each of the following items on a scale from 1–10.
These items may be completed by either the standardized patient or another student.

Scoresheet 1

	Poor		Fair		Good		Very Good		Excellent	
Professional appearance	1	2	3	4	5	6	7	8	9	10
Introduces self and shakes hands	1	2	3	4	5	6	7	8	9	10
Nonverbal communication (eye contact, facial expressiveness, body language)	1	2	3	4	5	6	7	8	9	10
Communicates effectively (open-ended questions, avoids jargon)	1	2	3	4	5	6	7	8	9	10
Establishes rapport with patient (empathy, appears nonjudgmental)	1	2	3	4	5	6	7	8	9	10
Allows patient to speak without being interrupted	1	2	3	4	5	6	7	8	9	10
Listens and seems to understand patient's concerns	1	2	3	4	5	6	7	8	9	10
Overall professionalism	1	2	3	4	5	6	7	8	9	10

Total Score:

Passing score for CIS section is 56 points.

Spoken English Proficiency (SEP) Scoresheet

Please rate each of the following items on a scale from 1–10.
These items may be completed by either the standardized patient or another student.

Scoresheet 2

	Poor		Fair		Good		Very Good		Excellent	
Examiner is articulate and easily understood	1	2	3	4	5	6	7	8	9	10
Pronunciation (words pronounced correctly; accent does not hinder communication)	1	2	3	4	5	6	7	8	9	10
Word choice is appropriate	1	2	3	4	5	6	7	8	9	10
Ability to communicate without excessive listener effort required to understand questions or responses	1	2	3	4	5	6	7	8	9	10
Patient's ability to understand the examiner	1	2	3	4	5	6	7	8	9	10
Examiner's ability to understand the patient	1	2	3	4	5	6	7	8	9	10

Total Score:

Passing score for SEP section is 42 points.

Standards for the Medical Care of the Adult Patient with Headache

Diagnosis

There are several important aspects to consider in the evaluation of the patient complaining of headache. As a priority, the clinician should consider the following:

1. Is there an acute emergency? Potentially worrisome features include the sudden onset of a severe headache (such as the so-called "thunderclap headache" indicating a subarachnoid hemorrhage), the presence of neurologic symptoms other than aura (such as weakness, numbness, paresthesias, speech difficulty, altered level of consciousness, ataxia, or seizure), the presence of focal or lateralizing neurologic deficits on exam, and associated constitutional symptoms such as fever, weight loss, or meningismus.
2. Is neuroimaging necessary? Although a patient's perception may differ, neuroimaging usually is not indicated. The majority of headache cases are indeed benign. Imaging is considered advisable for patients who have had any of the worrisome features mentioned in number one above. Neuroimaging may also be indicated for the patient who has had a new significant change in their headache pattern, known history of malignancy, age >50 and new onset or change in symptoms, recent head trauma, exertional or positional headaches, headache made worse by coughing or intercourse, or headache that awakens the patient from sleep. Immunocompromised patients and patients on anticoagulation medications also warrant special consideration.
3. Is specialty consultation appropriate? Some headache subtypes warrant assistance from a neurologist or headache specialist as the evaluation and management of certain headaches requires more training and expertise. These subtypes include refractory headache, frequent headaches that fail to respond to prophylaxis (see below), complicated migraine, trigeminal neuralgia, cluster headache, or any worrisome headache. Though consultation is not required for these subtypes of headache, it may be considered.

Common Primary Headache Subtypes

Migraine

Presentation: Mnemonic "SULTANS"

This type of headache is often defined by:

1. ***S***evere ***U***ni***L***ateral ***T***hrobbing pain made worse with physical ***A***ctivity
2. Associated with ***N***ausea and/or ***S***ensitivity to light or sound (photophobia and phonophobia)

Headache with at least two features from number one above and one symptom from number two could be considered migraine if there is no reason to suspect another cause. The presence or absence of a preceding aura, usually consisting of visual disturbances or scotomata, does not in itself make the diagnosis or rule out the diagnosis. Typically, migraines last 4 to 72 hours. Triggers include diet, emotional stress, menses, sleep deprivation, or changes in sleep patterns.

Treatment: The treatment of migraines can be divided into medications used to treat the acute headache (abortive) and agents used in their prevention (prophylaxis).

- Abortive agents include nonsteroidal anti-inflammatory drugs (NSAIDs) such as naproxen or ibuprofen combined with an antiemetic such as metoclopramide or prochlorperazine.
- Midrin and Cafergot have largely been replaced by the newer and more selective agents—the triptans.
- Sumatriptan (Imitrex), rizatriptan (Maxalt), and naratriptan (Amerge) are a few examples of this rapidly expanding class of medications. Their pharmacokinetics/pharmacodynamics vary widely.
- Dihydroergotamine (DHE) is also a valuable agent, especially to help abort a headache of prolonged duration.
- Prophylactic agents include tricyclic antidepressants such as amitriptyline or nortriptyline, β-blockers, calcium channel blockers, and anticonvulsants.

Episodic Tension Type

Presentation: These headaches are also quite common. Tension-type headaches are often described as a pressure, ache, tightness, or "band-like constriction" around the head. The severity of these symptoms does not generally influence the diagnosis. A stressful event may precipitate these headaches, as can the resolution of a stressful experience (the so-called "let down headache"). The absence of headache on vacation or weekends suggests tension type. Location of symptoms is commonly cervical, occipital, or temporal, though numerous variants exist. Palpation of these areas may reveal tender points or trigger points that reproduce headache symptoms. Nausea with or without vomiting may be associated.

Previously these headaches were thought to be caused by actual muscle tension leading to pain. More recently, as our understanding of headache pathophysiology advances, this subset is thought to exist along a continuum with migraine. It is common for patients to suffer from both. A patient with a predominance of tension-type symptoms along with several migraine features may be described as having a "migrainous" headache.

Treatment: Treatment of tension-type headache is very similar to migraine in both abortive and prophylaxis with the exception of triptans, which are used only for migraine headaches.

Analgesic Rebound

Presentation: Analgesic rebound headache should be high on the differential for a patient with chronic daily headaches. Often a patient begins with migraine or tension-type headaches on an episodic basis. With frequent use of analgesics, either over-the-counter or prescribed, patients begin to require more medication (both in dose and frequency of use). These headaches are then thought to "transform" into analgesic rebound if not managed appropriately. Previously called "drug rebound," as it was thought that potent narcotics were to blame, these headaches actually may be caused by any agent. Combination medications such as Excedrin (caffeine, aspirin, and acetaminophen) are often implicated.

Treatment: The treatment of analgesic rebound must be focused on removing the offending agent. Many patients are often switched to a prophylactic agent for long-term management, using transitional medications during the "weaning" process. Discontinuation of the analgesic requires thorough communication by the physician and clear understanding by the patient regarding what is causing the headaches. Transitional medications include longer-acting NSAIDS (piroxicam, nabumetone), triptans (naratriptan, frovatriptan, etc.), and in some cases, oral corticosteroids (Decadron).

Cluster Headache

Presentation: While much less common than the above types, cluster headaches may be quite incapacitating. These headaches often occur in attacks or clusters once or numerous times a day, with headache-free periods in between. Patients with cluster headaches often describe severe eye pain with associated lacrimation, redness, rhinorrhea, and nasal congestion.

Treatment: Medications sometimes used in the treatment of cluster headaches include indomethacin, methysergide, lithium carbonate, corticosteroids, sumatriptan, and DHE. Indomethacin is particularly effective in the treatment of chronic paroxysmal hemicrania, a subset of cluster headaches. Inhaled oxygen may also abort an acute attack. Prophylaxis may be achieved with various calcium channel blockers, divalproex, and topiramate often in combination with the above abortive agents.

Trigeminal Neuralgia (Tic Douloureux)

Presentation: Like cluster headaches, trigeminal neuralgia usually causes unilateral headache or facial pain. The two are often confused. Patients usually describe rapid paroxysms of burning or lancinating pain along the distribution of the involved trigeminal nerve branch. Stimulation of the face by rubbing, chewing, talking, and so forth can evoke attacks.

Treatment: As these symptoms are often quite severe, most first-line, low-potency analgesics are often ineffective. Anticonvulsants including carbamazepine, phenytoin, and gabapentin are commonly used therapeutic and/or prophylactic agents. Surgical or ablative treatment of the involved nerve branch should be considered for medication refractory cases.

Secondary Headaches

The list of potential sources of secondary headache is exhaustive. Brain tumor, subarachnoid hemorrhage, temporal arteritis, acute glaucoma, and acute bacterial meningitis should be considered, but their management would require interventions and treatment well beyond the scope of this exam. You should include these serious or potentially life-threatening conditions if asked to provide a differential diagnosis.

Key Physical Exam Points

- Vital signs are normal?
- Fever may indicate an infectious or inflammatory process

- Hypertension alone may cause headache but usually not until it is very high (systolic >200, diastolic >110). Headaches associated with associated tachycardia make pheochromocytoma a consideration.
- Normal eye exam, including the funduscopic exam for papilledema (indicating increased intracranial pressure), no Horner syndrome, no gaze diplopia, normal visual fields
- No temporal artery tenderness, swelling, or pulselessness
- Neck supple—no meningismus
- Neurologic exam normal—no gross focal or lateralizing deficits. This exam should include evaluation of cranial nerves, sensory perception, motor function, and gait.

REFERENCES

Bernat JL, Vincent FM. Neurology: Problems in Primary Care, 2nd ed. Los Angeles, Practice Management Information Corporation, 1993, pp 131–163.

Blau JN, Thavapala M. Preventing migraine: a study of precipitating factors. Headache 1988;28:481–483.

Capobianco DJ, Swanson JW, Dodick DW. Medication-induced (analgesic rebound) headache: Historical aspects and initial descriptions of the North American experience. Headache 2001;41(5):500–502.

Dodick D. Headache as a symptom of ominous disease. Postgrad Med 1997;101(5):46–64.

Featherstone HJ. Migraine and muscle contraction headache: A continuum. Headache 1985;25:194–198.

Headache Classification Committee of the International Headache Society. Classification and diagnostic criteria for headache disorders, cranial neuralgia, and facial pain. Cephalgia 1988;8(suppl 7):1–96.

Maizels M. The clinician's approach to the management of headache. West J Med 1998;168:203–212.

Spierings EL, Ranke AH, Honkoop PC. Precipitating and aggravating factors of migraine versus tension-type headache. Headache 2001;41:554–558.

"Our Baby Has a Fever"

Examinee Prompt

You are working in a pediatric urgent care clinic and are asked to see a 7-week-old infant for a chief complaint of fever. Please complete the following tasks:

- Obtain a thorough history from the parents of the patient.
- Perform an appropriate physical examination on the patient model. To receive credit, you will need to state out loud what specifically you are checking for (e.g., "I am checking the eardrums for redness or bulging").
- During this interaction, you may request any appropriate initial labs. The results of these tests will be provided to you by the parents.

You will have 15 minutes to complete the history and physical examination. When you have all of the information that you need, you may leave the examination room. Following your visit with the patient, you will be asked to write a complete progress note using the "SOAP" (Subjective, Objective, Assessment and Plan) format. You will have 10 additional minutes to complete this progress note.

Vital Signs

Temperature . . . . 38.7°C by rectal thermometer

Blood pressure 98/50

Heart rate 130

Respiratory rate 30

Weight . . . . 5.0 kg

Patient Prompt

Background: You will be playing the part of a worried parent. This is your first child who came after more than a year of infertility treatment. You have a sister who works as a nurse in a plastic surgery clinic. She has insisted that "a fever in a baby is a slam dunk admission to the hospital."

Chief Complaint: Fever

History of the Present Illness: This infant was the product of your first pregnancy at age 31. You had a normal spontaneous vaginal delivery of a vigorous baby at term (40 weeks). There were no complications of the pregnancy, labor, or delivery. There was no use of perinatal antibiotics and no history of group B streptococcus infection. After 2 days you brought your baby home and there were no concerns or problems. You saw a lactation consultant at a follow-up clinic 3 days after discharge (day 5 of life). There were no concerns at that time. There was no jaundice. At the 2-week visit and a 1-month well-child visit, there were no concerns by the doctor, though you and your spouse had numerous routine questions. Your child has never received antibiotics.

Over the last 2 days, you have noticed that your baby has been "much more fussy." For the past 24 hours, your child has had fevers, with a maximum rectal temperature of 38.7°C. These fevers are relieved with acetaminophen, but they return 6 to 8 hours later. There is some nasal congestion, but you were told this was normal. No cough, vomiting, or diarrhea. You have noted 6 to 8 wet diapers per day, which is unchanged since birth.

Past Medical History:
- Noncontributory, except as noted above.
- Weight gain has been appropriate.
- Birth weight was 3.5 kg.

Past Surgical History: None

Medications: Acetaminophen 80 mg orally every 4 to 8 hours

Allergies: No known drug allergies

Diet: Breast-fed ad-lib (usually 10 to 15 minutes on each breast every 3 to 6 hours)

Vaccination History: Hepatitis B at birth

Newborn Screening: All normal

Review of Symptoms: All development milestones met to date.
Otherwise negative except as noted above.

Additional Information: Obviously, it may be difficult to get an infant volunteer for this practice session. Please substitute a doll as the infant. As in reality, the infant actually offers very little in terms of history or complaint.

As the examiner performs the physical examination, he or she should state out loud what is being examined and why. As these statements are made, you may reply with the findings of the examination, which are provided in the "Objective" section of the scoring sheet. You should only respond to the portion of the examination that the examiner states out loud. For example, if the examiner states, "I am examining the anterior fontanel," you should state that "the anterior fontanelle is open and soft."

Infant With Fever Scoring Sheet

Subjective

- ❑ Asks chief complaint
- ❑ Duration of the fever
- ❑ Maximum temperature at home
- ❑ Asks how the temperature was taken (rectal, axillary, etc.)
- ❑ Response to antipyretics
- ❑ Asks about vomiting
- ❑ Asks about cough
- ❑ Asks about prenatal history
- ❑ Asks about method of delivery
- ❑ Birth weight
- ❑ Asks whether delivery was at term
- ❑ History of jaundice
- ❑ History of previous antibiotic administration
- ❑ History of any medical problems
- ❑ Hydration status, wet diapers per day

Objective

- ❑ General appearance: Awake and alert, no obvious distress. Good social smile, no respiratory distress.
- ❑ Hydration status: (Credit given if two of the following are examined): Mucous membranes are moist, the anterior fontanelle is open and soft, capillary refill is less than 2 seconds, skin color and turgor is normal.
- ❑ HEENT: Anterior fontanelle open and soft, tympanic membranes clear, oropharynx benign, nares show clear rhinorrhea
- ❑ Neck: No meningismus and no adenopathy
- ❑ Heart: Regular rate and rhythm, no murmurs
- ❑ Chest: Clear to auscultation bilaterally
- ❑ Abdomen: Soft, nontender, nondistended, normal bowel sounds
- ❑ Skin: No rash and no focal erythema; skin color and turgor are normal
- ❑ Extremities: No bony or soft-tissue erythema, swelling, or tenderness

Assessment

- ❑ Fever, rule out occult bacteremia

Plan

- ❑ Complete blood count (CBC)
- ❑ Urinalysis (must be a catheterized or suprapubic tap specimen)
- ❑ Chest x-ray
- ❑ Blood cultures
- ❑ Urine culture

Total Score: _____ / 30

Passing score for this station is 21 correct items.

Communication and Interpersonal Skills (CIS) Scoresheet

Please rate each of the following items on a scale from 1–10.
These items may be completed by either the standardized patient or another student.

Scoresheet 1

	Poor		Fair		Good		Very Good		Excellent	
Professional appearance	1	2	3	4	5	6	7	8	9	10
Introduces self and shakes hands	1	2	3	4	5	6	7	8	9	10
Nonverbal communication (eye contact, facial expressiveness, body language)	1	2	3	4	5	6	7	8	9	10
Communicates effectively (open-ended questions, avoids jargon)	1	2	3	4	5	6	7	8	9	10
Establishes rapport with patient (empathy, appears nonjudgmental)	1	2	3	4	5	6	7	8	9	10
Allows patient to speak without being interrupted	1	2	3	4	5	6	7	8	9	10
Listens and seems to understand patient's concerns	1	2	3	4	5	6	7	8	9	10
Overall professionalism	1	2	3	4	5	6	7	8	9	10

Total Score:

Passing score for CIS section is 56 points.

Spoken English Proficiency (SEP) Scoresheet

Please rate each of the following items on a scale from 1–10.
These items may be completed by either the standardized patient or another student.

Scoresheet 2

	Poor		Fair		Good		Very Good		Excellent	
Examiner is articulate and easily understood	1	2	3	4	5	6	7	8	9	10
Pronunciation (words pronounced correctly; accent does not hinder communication)	1	2	3	4	5	6	7	8	9	10
Word choice is appropriate	1	2	3	4	5	6	7	8	9	10
Ability to communicate without excessive listener effort required to understand questions or responses	1	2	3	4	5	6	7	8	9	10
Patient's ability to understand the examiner	1	2	3	4	5	6	7	8	9	10
Examiner's ability to understand the patient	1	2	3	4	5	6	7	8	9	10

Total Score:

Passing score for SEP section is 42 points.

MANAGEMENT OF THE FEBRILE INFANT

Overview

Over the last two decades, there has been a great deal of discussion regarding management of the febrile infant. Not long ago, all febrile infants under 8 weeks of age received cultures of the blood, urine, and spinal fluid, and were admitted for a sepsis evaluation. Over time, the age at which we automatically admitted patients was pushed back to 6 weeks. Very recently, some guidelines suggest that this age may be 4 weeks (28 days).

Some of the change in management is due to advancements in vaccination. Conjugated pneumococcal vaccine and *Haemophilus influenzae* (type B) vaccine have led to major changes in the field of pediatric infectious disease because of changes in the incidence of serious bacterial infection (SBI).

The major issue is in determining management is our ability to determine which infants are at significantly increased risk for SBI or occult bacteremia. We do know that younger infants, particularly those under 1 month of age, have less ability to contain and fight infections compared to their older cohorts. This places them at much higher risk for morbidity and mortality.

Serious Bacterial Infection

Because viral upper respiratory infections are so common, the parent and clinician may be inclined to attribute an infant's fever to "a cold or flu." However, the potential for SBI and its numerous serious complications must be considered, especially with younger infants.

Potential Sources for Serious Bacterial Infection

The four main sources for SBI are genitourinary (upper or lower urinary tract infection), blood-borne (bacteremia), respiratory (pneumonia), and central nervous system (meningitis). Infections of bone, soft tissue, and the gastrointestinal tract comprise a much less common group of sources.

Typical Pathogens

The most common pathogens in SBI include *Streptococcus* species (especially pneumococcus), *Haemophilus influenzae*, *Neisseria meningitidis*, *Salmonella* spp., *Escherichia coli*, *Enterococcus faecalis*, *Mycoplasma pneumoniae*, and *Listeria monocytogenes*.

The "Well-appearing" Child

The following discussion focuses on the infant less than 3 months of age. Children between 3 and 36 months of age typically are approached differently because of their more mature immune system as well as an improved ability on the part of the physician to determine which children appear clinically well and which children appear ill.

Several prospective trials in the literature (including Rochester, Boston, and Philadelphia) have looked at the management of the febrile infant and have proposed different criteria for establishing which children are at low risk for SBIs. Most of the difference of opinion on the topic of the febrile infant focuses on the appropriate management of a well-appearing, low-risk febrile infant. Rather than focus on the specific criteria in each of the studies, we feel that it is most helpful to understand which children are at low risk and know how to manage the febrile infant who may have occult bacteremia or an SBI.

The Yale Acute Illness Observation Scale (Table 1) provides a list of some observations that are pertinent to differentiating a well-appearing child from one who is ill. Much of this may seem intuitive, but nonetheless it is very important. It is vital to be able to articulate (and document) what specific factors lead you to the conclusion that a febrile infant is "well-appearing." Table 1 provides clinical signs that the physician may use to determine the current health status of a child.

Table 1

Yale Acute Illness Observation Scale

Strength/quality of cry	Reaction to parental stimulation
State variation (alertness)	Skin color
Hydration status	Response to social overtures

The "At-risk" Infant

The Rochester, Boston, and Philadelphia criteria often are used by clinicians to help identify which children are at an increased risk for developing SBI. In general, no single test or screening device can do this with 100% sensitivity or specificity. Unlike older patients that can offer some history, infants can harbor potentially life-threatening infections with fever as the only presenting symptom or sign.

There are numerous differences between the various study groups' recommendations, which may cause some confusion or frustration for medical students and house officers. By using the various available algorithms for evaluating the febrile infant, certain generalizations may be made. These general principles are as follows:

- Fever (defined as a rectal temperature of greater than 38°C) in a child age 28 days or less should prompt a full septic workup and admission to the hospital.
- In a child between 1 and 3 months of age, a screening CBC and urinalysis should be performed.
- Urine should be collected via suprapubic or urethral catheterization. Collection of urine in a bag is not considered to be an adequate specimen.
- If diarrhea is present, a microscopic examination of the stool should be included in this screening.
- Chest radiographs should be obtained if there are respiratory symptoms (cough, wheezing), respiratory distress (grunting, nasal flaring, retractions, tachypnea), hypoxia (SAO_2 < 95%), or abnormal respiratory sounds. With higher fevers (39.6°C or higher) or a white blood cell count (WBC) >20,000, many experts would recommend a chest radiograph even if the physical examination is normal.
- A child whose screening CBC, urinalysis, or chest radiograph is abnormal (Table 2) should be admitted and treated with intravenous antibiotics.
- Blood and urine cultures should be obtained in febrile children <12 weeks of age.

"Previously Healthy"

The Rochester criteria added the caveat that a child should be "previously healthy" to be managed within their guidelines. Although this makes intuitive sense in general, they were quite specific about which children should be considered. They are as follows:

- Born at term (>37 weeks)
- No history of perinatal antibiotics
- Discharged from hospital at the same time as mother
- Not treated for unexplained jaundice
- Has not received antibiotics and is not on antibiotics
- No previous hospitalization
- No chronic or underlying disease

Any child who does not meet these criteria should be considered to be at higher risk for an SBI, and should therefore be evaluated more thoroughly and aggressively.

Table 2

Screening Tests for the Workup of the Febrile Infant

Screening Test	Concerning Result
CBC	WBC >15,000 or <5000 *or* Bandemia >1500 *or* band-neutrophil ratio >0.2
UA	>10 WBC/hpf
CSF*	>6–10 WBC or Gram stain positive
CXR	Infiltrate present
Stool Micro (if diarrhea present)	Blood or >5 WBC/hpf

* There is some disagreement about which infants should undergo lumbar puncture. If a child is previously healthy, >8 weeks old, well appearing, and clinically has a respiratory tract infection with a normal CBC and CXR, bacterial meningitis is less likely. However, with younger patients, higher WBC, and higher fevers, CSF should be included in the screening evaluation. It is also reasonable to be more cautious with a child who has an incomplete vaccination history, or where follow-up may not be consistent.

CBC, complete blood count; CSF, cerebrospinal fluid; CXR, chest x-ray; hpf, high-power field; UA, urinalysis; WBC, white blood cell count.

Outpatient Management

Once the physician is satisfied that an infant is not at significantly increased risk for SBI, management may proceed on an outpatient basis. This means that the infant does not meet any of the criteria outlined in "the at-risk infant" above and does not have any of the concerning laboratory findings outlined in Table 2. For the patient being treated as an outpatient, there are several items to consider:

1. Make sure blood, urine (and cerebrospinal fluid if obtained) are sent for culture.
2. Arrange for follow-up within the next 24 hours.
3. Consider a single dose of parenteral ceftriaxone (50 to 75 mg/kg IM or IV) every 24 hours until urine and blood cultures have come back negative.
4. Treat fever with acetaminophen or ibuprofen (not aspirin due to the risk of Reye syndrome).
5. Encourage the parents to bring the child back for a repeat examination for any change in status or for any concern on the parents' part.

REFERENCES

Bachur RG, Harper MB. Predictive model for serious bacterial infections among infants younger than 3 months of age. Pediatrics 2001;108:311–316.

Baker MD, Bell LM, Avner JR. Outpatient management without antibiotics of fever in selected infants. N Engl J Med 1993;329:1437–1441.

Baraff LJ. Management of fever without source in infants and children. Ann Emerg Med 2000;36:602–614.

Baraff LJ, Bass JW, Fleisher GR, et al. Practice guideline for the management of infants and children 0 to 36 months of age with fever without source. Ann Emerg Med 1993;22:1198–1210.

Baskin MN, O'Rourke EJ, Fleisher GR. Outpatient treatment of febrile infants 28 to 89 days of age with intramuscular administration of ceftriaxone. J Pediatr 1992;120:22–27.

Bramson RT, Meyer TL, Silbiger ML, et al. The futility of the chest radiograph in the febrile infant without respiratory symptoms. Pediatrics 1993;92:524–526.

Jaskiewicz JA, McCarthy CA, Richardson AC, et al. Febrile infants at low risk for serious bacterial infection: An appraisal of the Rochester criteria and implications for management. Febrile Infant Collaborative Study Group. Pediatrics 1994;94:390–396.

Luszczak M. Evaluation and management of infants and young children with fever. Am Fam Physician 2001;64(7):1219–1226.

"My Cold Won't Go Away"

Examinee Prompt

You are seeing this 42-year-old woman in your office for a chief complaint of "cough." Please complete the following tasks:

- Obtain a focused history relevant to this patient's complaint.
- Conduct an appropriate physical examination.
- Outline a course of treatment for the patient, as well as follow-up, if necessary.

You have 15 minutes to complete your visit with the patient. When you have all of the information that you need you may leave the examination room. Following your visit with the patient, you will be asked to write a progress using the standard "SOAP" (Subjective, Objective, Assessment and Plan) format. You will have 10 additional minutes to complete the progress note.

Vital Signs

Temperature .... 99.0°F

Blood pressure 132/80

Pulse 78

Respiratory rate 16

Patient Prompt

Background: You are a 42-year-old patient complaining of a cough for about 3 months.

Chief Complaint: Cough

History of the Present Illness: 42-year-old woman with a 3-month history of non-productive cough. The cough began as "a regular cold," but the cough has persisted after the other cold symptoms resolved. The cough is more troublesome at night. Friends and coworkers have commented on the cough, which is what motivated the visit today. The coughing occurs in "fits" triggered by cold air, laughing, or prolonged talking. (As the standardized patient, you should only offer the triggers if specifically asked.)

Past Medical History: Bronchitis as a child

Past Surgical History: Tonsillectomy age 8, appendectomy age 14

Gynecologic History: G2 P2, two normal spontaneous vaginal deliveries

Medications: Oral contraceptive pills

Allergies: Sulfa medication caused a rash in the past

Family History:
- Father died of pancreatic cancer at age 67
- Mother living, age 70, with a history of hypertension and hyperlipidemia
- Siblings are healthy

Social History:
- Married for 17 years
- 2 children
- Works as an administrative assistant in a large corporation
- Tobacco use 1/2 pack per day for 12 years
- Your husband smokes as well
- Drinks approximately 3 glasses of wine per week
- Exercises at the gym 4 times per week
- No pets or recent travel

Review of Systems:
- No fevers, no chest pain, no shortness of breath, no audible wheezing, no hemoptysis
- No gastroesophageal reflux disease (GERD) symptoms (no heartburn, no metallic or sour taste in the mouth)
- No postnasal drip or rhinorrhea
- On two occasions there has been posttussive emesis
- Review of systems is otherwise negative

Additional Information: The examination results are unremarkable.

Chronic Cough Scoring Sheet

Subjective

- ❑ Duration of cough
- ❑ Productive or nonproductive cough
- ❑ Tobacco use
- ❑ Fever
- ❑ Shortness of breath
- ❑ Chest pain
- ❑ Wheezing
- ❑ Triggers
- ❑ GERD symptoms
- ❑ Postnasal drip/rhinorrhea
- ❑ Hemoptysis
- ❑ Past medical history
- ❑ History of asthma
- ❑ Family history
- ❑ Pets
- ❑ Travel history

Objective

- ❑ Lymphadenopathy
- ❑ Oropharynx
- ❑ Nasal passages
- ❑ Pulmonary exam
- ❑ Abdominal exam

Diagnosis

- ❑ Asthma (or specifically cough-variant asthma) included in differential diagnosis
- ❑ Chronic bronchitis included in differential diagnosis

Plan

- ❑ Chest x-ray
- ❑ Pulse oximetry
- ❑ Smoking cessation recommended
- ❑ Pulmonary function tests ordered
- ❑ Follow-up plan outlined

Total Score: _____ / 28

Passing score for this station is 19 correct items.

Communication and Interpersonal Skills (CIS) Scoresheet

Please rate each of the following items on a scale from 1–10.
These items may be completed by either the standardized patient or another student.

Scoresheet 1

	Poor		Fair		Good		Very Good		Excellent	
Professional appearance	1	2	3	4	5	6	7	8	9	10
Introduces self and shakes hands	1	2	3	4	5	6	7	8	9	10
Nonverbal communication (eye contact, facial expressiveness, body language)	1	2	3	4	5	6	7	8	9	10
Communicates effectively (open-ended questions, avoids jargon)	1	2	3	4	5	6	7	8	9	10
Establishes rapport with patient (empathy, appears nonjudgmental)	1	2	3	4	5	6	7	8	9	10
Allows patient to speak without being interrupted	1	2	3	4	5	6	7	8	9	10
Listens and seems to understand patient's concerns	1	2	3	4	5	6	7	8	9	10
Overall professionalism	1	2	3	4	5	6	7	8	9	10

Total Score:

Passing score for CIS section is 56 points.

Spoken English Proficiency (SEP) Scoresheet

Please rate each of the following items on a scale from 1–10.
These items may be completed by either the standardized patient or another student.

Scoresheet 2

	Poor		Fair		Good		Very Good		Excellent	
Examiner is articulate and easily understood	1	2	3	4	5	6	7	8	9	10
Pronunciation (words pronounced correctly; accent does not hinder communication)	1	2	3	4	5	6	7	8	9	10
Word choice is appropriate	1	2	3	4	5	6	7	8	9	10
Ability to communicate without excessive listener effort required to understand questions or responses	1	2	3	4	5	6	7	8	9	10
Patient's ability to understand the examiner	1	2	3	4	5	6	7	8	9	10
Examiner's ability to understand the patient	1	2	3	4	5	6	7	8	9	10

Total Score:

Passing score for SEP section is 42 points.

Approach to the Patient With Chronic Cough

Differential Diagnosis

Cough may be characterized based upon duration. An acute cough lasts less than 3 weeks. Subacute cough lasts 3 to 8 weeks. Chronic cough persists beyond 8 weeks.

The differential diagnosis of cough is guided by the chronicity of the cough. The differential diagnosis of each type of cough is provided below.

Acute Cough

- Viral upper respiratory tract infection (the most common cause of acute cough)
- Allergic rhinitis
- Acute bacterial sinusitis
- Acute exacerbation of chronic obstructive pulmonary disease (COPD)
- Pertussis infection
- Environmental exposures such as tobacco smoke, dust

Subacute Cough

- Most cases of subacute cough result from bacterial sinusitis or asthma
- Upper respiratory tract infection
- Pertussis infection (can be acute or subacute)

Chronic Cough

There are three causes of chronic cough that account for most cases, and these three causes are commonly referred to as the "pathogenic triad of chronic cough." In order, these causes are:

1. Postnasal drip syndrome
2. Asthma
3. GERD

Evaluating the Patient with Chronic Cough

Any evaluation of chronic cough should begin with a thorough medical history and physical examination. Areas of particular interest in the medical history include tobacco smoking, environmental exposures, animal exposures, travel history, and treatments rendered prior to the evaluation. Angiotensin-converting enzyme (ACE) inhibitors cause a nonproductive cough in 5% to 20% of persons taking them and should be considered in any person with a chronic cough. The cough may begin several days to several months after the medication is started.

The review of systems may provide useful information regarding the etiology of the cough. Throat clearing or a complaint of nasal congestion may suggest the presence of postnasal drip syndrome. Wheezing or cough may suggest asthma as the cause of chronic cough. Coughing alone is the only manifestation of asthma (cough-variant asthma) in up to 57% of patients with the disease. Cough-variant asthma should be considered when chronic cough is exacerbated by cold or exercise, or when the cough worsens at night. Complaints of heartburn, regurgitation, and bloating may suggest a GERD-induced chronic cough. However, GERD may be clinically silent yet produce a chronic cough. Postinfectious cough should be considered when cough persists after an upper respiratory tract infection.

A chest radiograph generally is recommended in the initial evaluation of the chronic cough. A normal chest radiograph usually excludes malignancy, bronchiectasis, persistent pneumonia, sarcoidosis, and tuberculosis as the cause of the cough. There are, however, several situations in which a chest radiograph is optional in the initial evaluation of chronic cough:

- If a patient is taking an ACE inhibitor, a trial off this medication is reasonable before a chest radiograph is obtained. The cough should subside several days to several weeks after the ACE inhibitor is discontinued. If the cough persists, a chest radiograph should be obtained.
- In younger nonsmokers in whom postnasal drip syndrome or sinusitis is suspected, a chest radiograph may be deferred. However, if the cough persists after adequate treatment for the suspected disorder, a chest radiograph should be obtained.
- In pregnant women with chronic cough, the chest radiograph is not required.

If the chest radiograph is abnormal, further evaluation may be warranted. Additional studies depend upon the suspected diagnosis but may include computed tomography (CT) scanning of the chest, bronchoscopy, barium esophagography, or pulmonary function tests.

If the chest radiograph is normal, the next step is to consider the patient's symptom complex and history to determine which of the common causes may be the most likely diagnosis. In the absence of one diagnosis that is most likely, the three most common diagnoses may be treated empirically one at a time in order of likelihood. For each of the conditions, 2 weeks of therapy is usually sufficient before the next most likely cause is considered. These conditions are outlined in Tables 1 and 2.

Table 1

Causes of Chronic Cough in Adults

Common Causes	Less Common Causes	Uncommon Causes
Postnasal drip syndrome Asthma Gastroesophageal reflux disease Angiotensin-converting enzyme inhibitors Smoking and other irritants Bronchitis	Pertussis infection Bronchiectasis Eosinophilic bronchitis Postinfectious	Aspiration Bronchogenic carcinoma Carcinomatosis Irritable larynx Lymphoma Persistent pneumonia Psychogenic cough Pulmonary abscess Sarcoidosis Tuberculosis

Table 2

Causes of Chronic Cough in Children

Common Causes	Less Common Causes	Uncommon Causes
Upper and lower respiratory tract infections Gastroesophageal reflux disease	Foreign body aspiration	Congenital abnormality Cystic fibrosis Environmental exposures Immunologic disorder Primary ciliary dyskinesia Psychogenic cough Tourette syndrome Tuberculosis

Causes of Chronic Cough

Postnasal Drip Syndrome

Presentation: Alone or in combination with other conditions, postnasal drip syndrome is the most common cause of chronic cough in nonsmoking, immunocompetent adults. As such, it is often the first condition to be treated empirically. *Postnasal drip syndrome* is a term that encompasses multiple clinical entities including allergic rhinitis, vasomotor rhinitis, and sinusitis.

Though no signs or symptoms are specific to cough caused by postnasal drip, certain symptoms and signs may suggest this diagnosis. Frequent throat clearing, sore throat, a history of allergies, and a "cobblestone" appearance of the posterior pharynx are features that suggest the diagnosis of postnasal drip syndrome.

Examination: Radiography of the sinuses may be considered when sinusitis is suspected as the cause of postnasal drip syndrome. However, sinus radiographs are neither sensitive nor specific for the diagnosis of sinusitis.

Treatment: Postnasal drip syndrome suspected to be caused by sinusitis should be treated appropriately with decongestants with or without antibiotics. Postnasal drip syndrome not caused by sinusitis usually responds to treatment with a decongestant and a first-generation H_1 antihistamine. If allergic rhinitis is suspected, a nasal steroid is appropriate. If vasomotor rhinitis is suspected as the cause, nasal ipratropium bromide is the preferred treatment.

Asthma

Presentation: Asthma is the second most common cause of chronic cough after postnasal drip syndrome. Though asthma is often considered in patients with a history of wheezing or shortness of breath, coughing is the only manifestation of asthma in up to 57% of patients with the disease (cough-variant asthma). Cough-variant asthma should be considered in the patient whose chronic cough is worsened by cold or exercise. These patients often report a cough that worsens at night.

Examination: A methacholine challenge test is recommended in patients in whom cough-variant asthma is suspected because a negative result essentially rules out asthma as the cause of chronic cough.

Treatment: Cough-variant asthma usually is treated with inhaled corticosteroids and bronchodilators.

GERD

Presentation: GERD is the third most common cause of chronic cough in immunocompetent, nonsmoking adults. Though complaints of heartburn, gassiness, bloating, and regurgitation suggest the diagnosis of GERD as the cause of chronic cough, GERD may also be clinically silent with the exception of the chronic cough.

Examination: No specific study is recommended in the routine evaluation of GERD.

Treatment: An empiric treatment of antireflux medication such as a proton pump inhibitor or an H_2 antihistamine is instead suggested.

Chronic Bronchitis

Presentation: Chronic bronchitis from exposure to cigarette smoking or other environmental irritants is a common cause of chronic cough. However, many persons with smoker's cough do not seek medical care, perhaps because they accept the cough as an effect of smoking.

Examination: A chest radiograph and pulmonary function tests may be considered. In refractory cases, bronchoscopy sometimes is performed.

Treatment: The principle of treatment in these patients is to eliminate tobacco smoke or the offending environmental irritant.

Eosinophilic Bronchitis

Presentation: Eosinophilic bronchitis has only recently been reported as a cause of chronic cough, yet it has been found in 10% to 20% of patients referred to pulmonary medicine clinics for evaluation of their cough.

Examination: Eosinophils and metachromatic cells in the sputum differentiate eosinophilic bronchitis from chronic bronchitis.

Treatment: These patients respond to inhaled and systemic corticosteroids.

Postinfectious Cough

Presentation: Postinfectious cough should be considered in any patient whose cough persists following an upper respiratory tract infection.

Examination: No specific studies are necessary for this cause.

Treatment: This cough will eventually resolve without treatment. However, inhaled ipratropium bromide (Atrovent), inhaled corticosteroids, or oral corticosteroids may hasten resolution of symptoms.

Pertussis

Presentation: Pertussis infection in the adolescent and adult population has been on the rise, most likely due to an increased recognition and diagnosis of pertussis among age groups beyond childhood. Pertussis infection typically begins with a catarrhal stage consisting of rhinorrhea and mild cough which can last up to 2 weeks. This is followed by paroxysms of irritating cough that initially is dry but becomes productive of clear, tenacious mucus. Prolonged paroxysms of coughing can be associated with vomiting or syncope. The paroxysmal stage is followed by up to 2 months of cough that can disturb sleep.

Examination: Pertussis in adolescents and adults can be diagnosed by bacterial culture, polymerase chain reaction (PCR), or by serologic methods. Most authors agree in recommending the use of *Bordetella*-PCR in combination with serology to diagnose pertussis in adolescents and adults.

Treatment: Pertussis is treated with a 14-day course of either erythromycin or trimethoprim-sulfamethoxazole.

Bronchogenic Carcinoma

Presentation: Bronchogenic carcinoma is much more likely in patients who smoke or who have a smoking history, but does occur in nonsmokers as well.

Examination: In the patient who smokes, a chest radiograph should be included as part of the initial evaluation of the chronic cough. If the findings of the chest radiograph are suspicious for malignancy, CT scanning should be performed.

Treatment: If the chest radiograph is normal but symptoms persist despite a thorough evaluation for the other common causes of chronic cough, CT scanning of the chest and referral to a pulmonologist for bronchoscopy should be considered.

Bronchiectasis

Presentation: Bronchiectasis is an infrequent cause of chronic cough characterized by overproduction of sputum, fever, pleurisy, and malodorous or blood-tinged sputum. Bronchiectasis should be considered in any patient in whom chronic cough produces sputum and hemoptysis.

Examination: The chest radiograph is usually abnormal in patients with bronchiectasis, but CT scanning of the chest is considered the gold standard for diagnosing bronchiectasis.

Treatment: A patient in whom bronchiectasis is considered should be referred to a pulmonologist.

Psychogenic Cough

Presentation: Psychogenic cough is a diagnosis that should be made only after all other possibilities have been eliminated. Psychogenic cough occurs more commonly in children than in adults. Psychogenic cough is characterized by a cough that does not occur during sleep, does not awaken the patient from sleep, and usually does not occur during enjoyable distractions.

Examination: Psychogenic cough may be exacerbated by psychologic stressors.

Treatment: Psychogenic cough is treated by minimizing psychological stressors and through behavioral modification therapy.

REFERENCES

Brightling CE, Ward R, Wardlaw AJ, Pavord ID. Airway inflammation, airway responsiveness and cough before and after inhaled budesonide in patients with eosinophilic bronchitis. Eur Respir J 2000;15:682–686.

Brightling CE, Ward R, Goh KL, Wardlaw AJ, Pavord ID. Eosinophilic bronchitis is an important cause of chronic cough. Am J Respir Crit Care Med 1999;160:406–410.

Gonzales R, Bartlett JG, Besser RE, et al. Principles of appropriate antibiotic use for treatment of uncomplicated acute bronchitis: Background. Ann Emerg Med 2001;37:720–727.

Haber LR, Waseem M, Basnight LL, et al. Index of suspicion. Pediatr Rev 2002;23:179–185.

Hogan MB, Wilson NW. Tourette's syndrome mimicking asthma. J Asthma 1999;36:253–256.

Holmes RL, Fadden CT. Evaluation of the patient with chronic cough. Am Fam Physician 2004;69: 2159–2168.

Hoey J. Pertussis in adults. Can Med Assoc J 2003;168:453–454.

Irwin RS, Boulet LP, Cloutier MM, et al. Managing cough as a defense mechanism and as a symptom. A consensus panel report of the American College of Chest Physicians. Chest 1998;114(2 suppl) 133S–181S.

Irwin RS, Madison JM. The diagnosis and treatment of cough. N Engl J Med 2000;343:1715–1721.

Karras DJ. Update on emerging infections: News from the Centers for Disease Control and Prevention. Ann Emerg Med 2002;40:115–119.

Mello CJ, Irwin RS, Curley FJ. Predictive values of the character, timing, and complications of chronic cough in diagnosing its cause. Arch Intern Med 1996;156:997–1003.

Mysliwiec V, Pina JS. Bronchiectasis: The "other" obstructive lung disease. Postgrad Med 1999;106: 123–6,128–131.

Ours TM, Kavuru MS, Schilz RJ, Richter JE. A prospective evaluation of esophageal testing and a double-blind, randomized study of omeprazole in a diagnostic and therapeutic algorithm for chronic cough. Am J Gastroenterol 1999;94:3131–3138.

Palombini BC, Villanova CA, Araujo E, et al. A pathogenic triad in chronic cough: Asthma, postnasal drip syndrome, and gastroesophageal reflux disease. Chest 1999;116:279–284.

Wirsing von Konig CH, Halperin S, Riffelman M, Guiso N. Pertussis of adults and infants. Lancet 2002;2:744–750.

“My Knee Popped”

Examinee Prompt

You are seeing this 19-year-old woman in your office for a chief complaint of "knee pain." Please complete the following tasks:

- Obtain a focused history relevant to this patient's complaint.
- Perform an appropriate physical examination.
- Outline a course of treatment for the patient, as well as follow-up, if necessary.

You have 15 minutes to complete your visit with the patient. When you have all of the information that you will need, you may leave the examination room. Following your visit with the patient, you will be asked to generate a differential diagnosis as well as a treatment plan. In this station, you will be asked to write a complete progress note using the standard SOAP (Subjective, Objective, Assessment and Plan) format. You will have 10 additional minutes to complete this portion of the progress note.

Patient Prompt

Background: You are a 19-year-old collegiate soccer player with a concern about pain in your left knee that began when you planted your foot awkwardly while kicking a soccer ball.

Chief Complaint: Left knee pain

History of the Present Illness: 19-year-old collegiate soccer player who had immediate onset of left knee pain that occurred when the foot was planted awkwardly while kicking a soccer ball. The pain was sufficient that the patient was unable to return to the playing field. The knee does sometimes click and gives a locking sensation when complete extension is attempted. The knee has the sensation that it is going to give way, though weight-bearing is possible. There has been mild swelling of the knee.

Past Medical History: None. No previous history of knee trauma

Past Surgical History: None. No previous knee surgeries

Gynecologic History: G0. Unremarkable gynecologic history

Medications: None

Allergies: No known drug allergies

Family History: Unremarkable family history

Social History:
- 19-year-old college student who plays varsity soccer
- Single, no children
- No tobacco, alcohol, or drug use

Review of Systems: Unremarkable except as outlined in the history of the present illness

Additional Information: Please study the examination section of this chapter before acting as the standardized patient. You should understand the examination of the knee well in order to tell the examiner what portions of the examination cause you pain.

During the examination, the following are pertinent positives:
- You should act as though there is tenderness along the medial joint line.
- Complete flexion causes you pain.
- You are unable to complete a deep knee bend because of discomfort.
- McMurray test is positive.

Scoring Sheet

Subjective

- ❑ Onset/duration of pain
- ❑ Location of pain
- ❑ Severity of pain
- ❑ Quality of pain
- ❑ History of trauma to the knee
- ❑ Exacerbating and alleviating factors
- ❑ Swelling
- ❑ Clicking or locking
- ❑ Sensation of instability
- ❑ Previous knee problems or knee surgery

Objective

- ❑ Visual inspection of the knee
- ❑ Palpation of major structures (at least four of the following: patella, medial joint line, lateral joint line, popliteal fossa, tibial tubercle, patellar tendon, quadriceps tendon)
- ❑ Range of motion
- ❑ Patellar compression test
- ❑ Anterior drawer test
- ❑ Valgus stress test
- ❑ Varus stress test
- ❑ McMurray test or deep knee bend

Assessment (these two items should be included in the differential diagnosis)

- ❑ Meniscal tear
- ❑ Medial collateral ligament sprain

Plan

- ❑ Ice
- ❑ Rest with immobilization
- ❑ Analgesics or anti-inflammatory medication
- ❑ Follow-up if not improved in 4 to 8 weeks

Total Score: _____ / 24

Passing score for this station is 16 correct items.

Communication and Interpersonal Skills (CIS) Scoresheet

Please rate each of the following items on a scale from 1–10.
These items may be completed by either the standardized patient or another student.

Scoresheet 1

	Poor		Fair		Good		Very Good		Excellent	
Professional appearance	1	2	3	4	5	6	7	8	9	10
Introduces self and shakes hands	1	2	3	4	5	6	7	8	9	10
Nonverbal communication (eye contact, facial expressiveness, body language)	1	2	3	4	5	6	7	8	9	10
Communicates effectively (open-ended questions, avoids jargon)	1	2	3	4	5	6	7	8	9	10
Establishes rapport with patient (empathy, appears nonjudgmental)	1	2	3	4	5	6	7	8	9	10
Allows patient to speak without being interrupted	1	2	3	4	5	6	7	8	9	10
Listens and seems to understand patient's concerns	1	2	3	4	5	6	7	8	9	10
Overall professionalism	1	2	3	4	5	6	7	8	9	10

Total Score:

Passing score for CIS section is 56 points.

Spoken English Proficiency (SEP) Scoresheet

Please rate each of the following items on a scale from 1–10.
These items may be completed by either the standardized patient or another student.

Scoresheet 2

	Poor		Fair		Good		Very Good		Excellent	
Examiner is articulate and easily understood	1	2	3	4	5	6	7	8	9	10
Pronunciation (words pronounced correctly; accent does not hinder communication)	1	2	3	4	5	6	7	8	9	10
Word choice is appropriate	1	2	3	4	5	6	7	8	9	10
Ability to communicate without excessive listener effort required to understand questions or responses	1	2	3	4	5	6	7	8	9	10
Patient's ability to understand the examiner	1	2	3	4	5	6	7	8	9	10
Examiner's ability to understand the patient	1	2	3	4	5	6	7	8	9	10

Total Score:

Passing score for SEP section is 42 points.

Approach to the Patient With Knee Pain

History

The evaluation of acute or chronic knee pain begins with a thorough history. The patient's description of the knee pain can be helpful in focusing the differential diagnosis and guiding the evaluation. The following historical items should be obtained:

1. Duration and location of the pain
2. Onset of pain (rapid or insidious)
3. Precipitating and alleviating factors
4. Location of pain
5. Severity
6. Quality (sharp, dull, achy)
7. Recent or previous injury. If so, what was the mechanism of injury? If the knee pain is caused by an acute injury, inquire whether the patient was able to continue activity or bear weight after the injury.
    - Direct lateral force applied to the outside of the knee can result in rupture of the medial collateral ligament (MCL), rupture of the anterior cruciate ligament (ACL), and a torn meniscus (the so-called "unhappy triad").
    - A force applied medially can injure the lateral collateral ligament.
    - A direct blow applied anteriorly to the proximal tibia with the knee in flexion, as may occur when the knee strikes the dashboard in an automobile accident, can injure the posterior cruciate ligament (PCL).
    - Quick stops and sharp turns can sprain or rupture the ACL.
    - Sudden twisting or pivoting motions can result in meniscal tear.
    - Hyperextension may injure the ACL or PCL.
8. Swelling. Onset of swelling within 2 hours after injury is a sign of hemarthrosis, which suggests rupture of the ACL or fracture of the tibial plateau. An effusion with a slower onset suggests a meniscal injury or ligamentous strain. Recurrent knee effusion after activity suggests an intra-articular lesion irritating the synovium, such as a meniscal tear.
9. Locking. A knee that locks cannot be fully extended and suggests a meniscal tear. This must be differentiated from a knee that cannot be fully extended due to pain or swelling.
10. Clicking or catching. Recurrent clicking or catching can be due to a torn meniscus, loose body, or degenerative arthritis.
11. Knee instability or a sensation of the knee giving way suggests patellar subluxation or ligamentous rupture, but may also be due to a torn meniscus or osteochondritis desiccans. Patellofemoral pain or degenerative arthritis may cause the knee to intermittently give way.
12. Grating sensations are common with degenerative arthritis and patellofemoral pain.
13. Other joint involvement may suggest gout or rheumatologic processes.
14. Ask about previous knee problems or surgery.

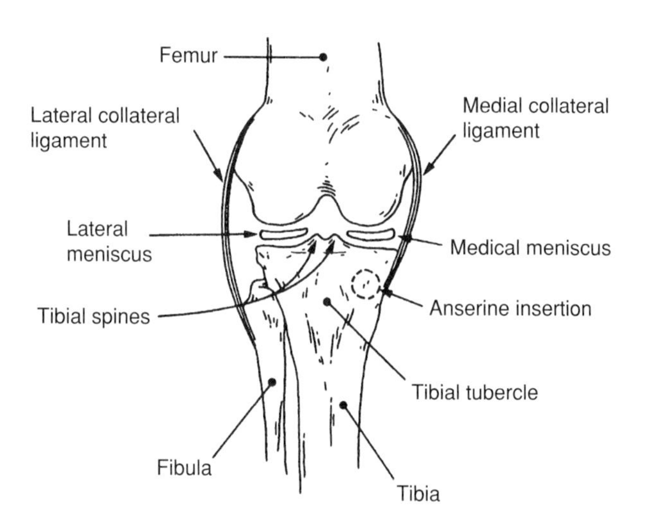

Figure 1. Anatomy of the knee anterior **(A)** and lateral **(B)** views

Examination

The examination of the knee begins with visual inspection (Figure 1). The injured knee should be examined for erythema, swelling, and bruising. Following visual inspection, the knee should be palpated for tenderness, warmth, or effusion. The following structures should be palpated individually for point tenderness:

- Patella
- Patellar tendon (Figure 2A)
- Tibial tubercle (Figure 2B)
- Quadriceps tendon
- Medial joint line (Figure 3A)
- Lateral joint line
- Anteromedial joint line
- Anterolateral joint line

Assess muscle tone by measuring thigh circumference approximately 6 cm above the top of the patella. More than 1 cm difference between the two thighs is significant and indicates a true problem with the involved leg. The tone of the contracted quadriceps should also be evaluated to determine whether atrophy is present.

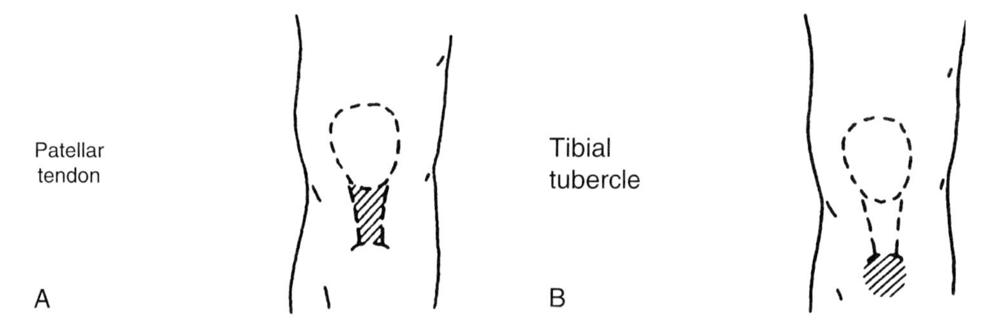

Figure 2. Patellar tendon **(A)** and tibial tubercle **(B)**. Tenderness along the patellar tendon usually indicates patellar tendonitis. However, tenderness at the inferior aspect of the tendon over the tibial tubercle in an adolescent suggests Osgood-Schlatter disease.

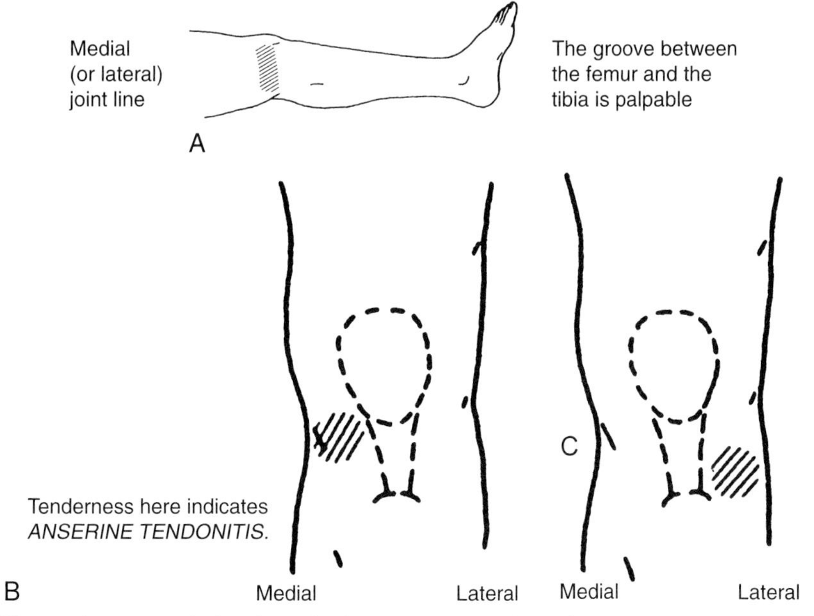

Figure 3. **(A)** Medial or lateral joint line. The location of tenderness along the joint line may help in determining the etiology of knee pain. In degenerative arthritis, joint line tenderness tends to be diffuse. In meniscal injury, the point of maximal tenderness migrates slightly posteriorly as the knee is flexed. In ligamentous injury, tenderness usually extends a bit above the joint line. **(B)** The anserine tendons insert at the anteromedial aspect of the proximal tibia, just inferior to the medial joint line. Tenderness at this point indicates pes anserine bursitis (also called pes anserine tendonitis). **(C)** Tenderness over the anterolateral tibia indicates iliotibial band tendonitis.

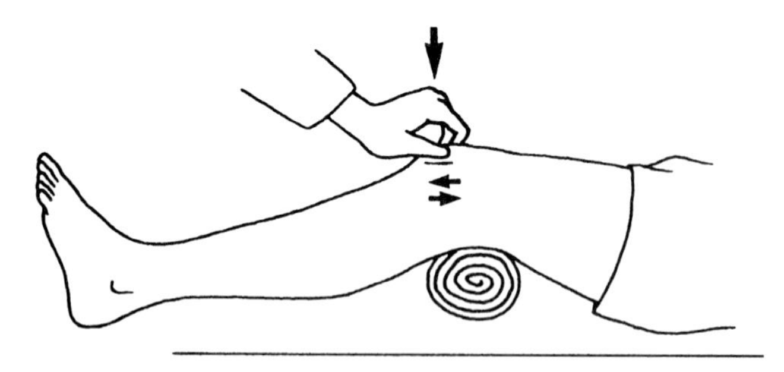

Figure 4. Patellar Compression Test. The patella is moved proximally and distally as downward compression is applied. Pain or crepitus is a positive test, implying patellofemoral pain syndrome (also called chondromalacia in the younger patient and implying degenerative arthritis of the patellofemoral joint in the older patient).

Following visual inspection and palpation, range of motion should be assessed. Normal range of motion is extension to zero degrees and flexion to 135 degrees. If there is any limitation in range of motion, it should be determined whether a true limitation exists or whether the limitation is due to pain or effusion.

Each of the major structures should then be assessed. The major structures are outlined below, along with the appropriate tests.

Patellofemoral Assessment

- Tenderness over patellar tendon
- Patellar compression test (Figure 4)
- Patellar apprehension test (Figure 5)

Anterior Cruciate Ligament

- Anterior drawer test (Figure 6A, B)
- Lachman test (Figure 7)

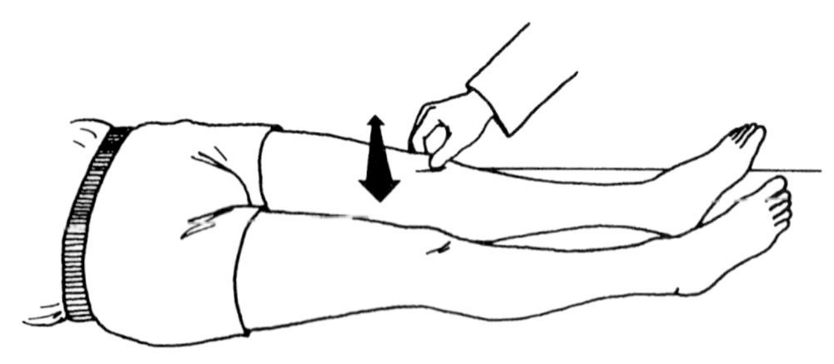

Figure 5. Patellar Apprehension Test. The patient is asked to relax the muscles. The examiner's fingers are placed at the medial aspect of the patella, and the examiner attempts to sublux the patella laterally. The test is considered positive if the maneuver reproduces the patient's pain, if the patient resists, or if the test produces a sensation that the patella is going to give way. A positive test suggests patellar subluxation as the diagnosis.

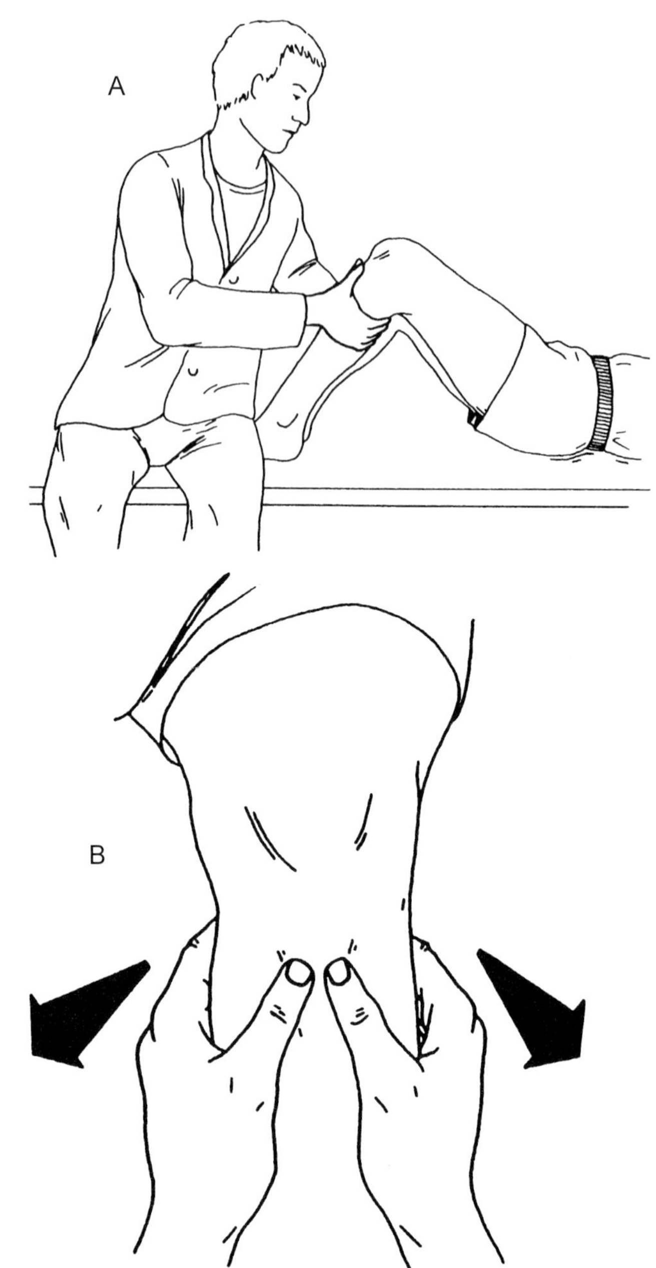

Figure 6. *(Continued)*

Posterior Cruciate Ligament

- Posterior drawer test (Figure 6C)

Medial Collateral Ligament

- Tenderness over MCL
- Valgus stress test (Figure 8)

Lateral Collateral Ligament

- Tenderness over lateral collateral ligament
- Varus stress test (Figure 9)

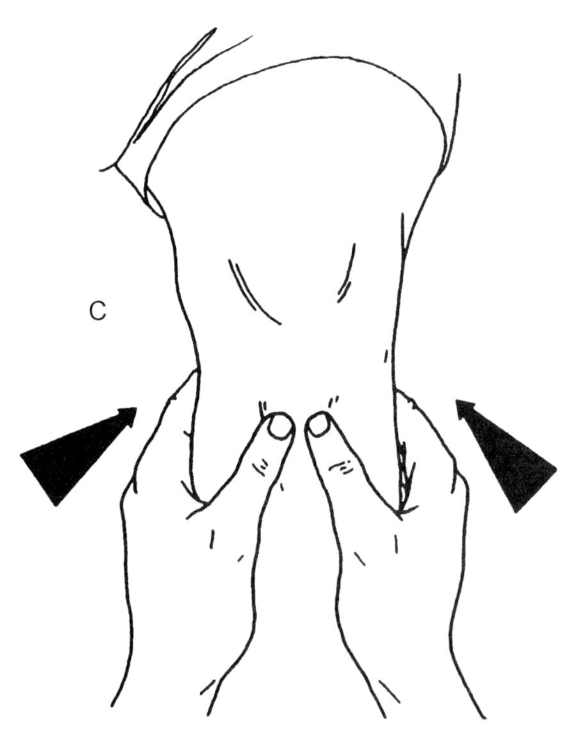

Figure 6. **(A)** The drawer tests evaluate the integrity of the anterior cruciate ligament (ACL) and the posterior cruciate ligament (PCL). The patient is placed in the supine position, and the injured knee is flexed to 90 degrees. The examiner sits on the patient's foot to fix it in place while placing both thumbs at the tibial tubercle and fingers at the posterior calf. **(B)** Anterior drawer test. The patient is asked to relax the hamstring muscles while the examiner pulls anteriorly. The uninvolved knee is likewise examined, and an asymmetric laxity indicates a torn ACL. **(C)** Posterior drawer test. The examiner pushes posteriorly. Posterior displacement of the tibia suggests a torn ACL.

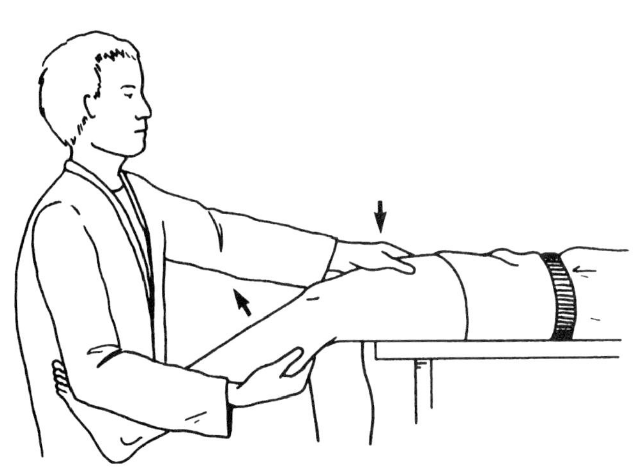

Figure 7. Lachman Test. The Lachman test helps assess the integrity of the ACL. The patient is placed in the supine position and the knee is flexed to 30 degrees. The distal femur is stabilized with one hand while the proximal tibia is grasped posteriorly with the other hand. The examiner then attempts to sublux the tibia anteriorly. The lack of a clear end point represents a positive Lachman test and indicates an ACL rupture. Comparison should be made with the uninvolved side to ensure an accurate result.

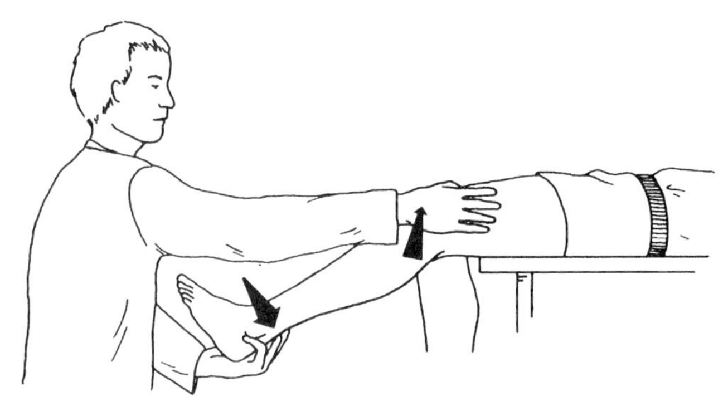

Figure 8. Valgus Stress Test. The valgus stress test assesses the integrity of the medial collateral ligament. The patient is placed in the supine position. The examiner places one hand at the lateral aspect of the knee joint and the other hand at the heel. The patient's knee is flexed to 30 degrees and valgus stress is applied to assess stability of the medial collateral ligament. The injured knee should be compared to the uninvolved knee.

Menisci

- Tenderness over the medial or lateral joint line
- McMurray test (Figure 10)
- Deep knee bend

Posterior Knee

- Evaluation for a Baker cyst

Specific Causes of Knee Pain

Anterior Cruciate Ligament Injury

Presentation: ACL injuries most often occur with forces such as landing hard on a slightly flexed knee,

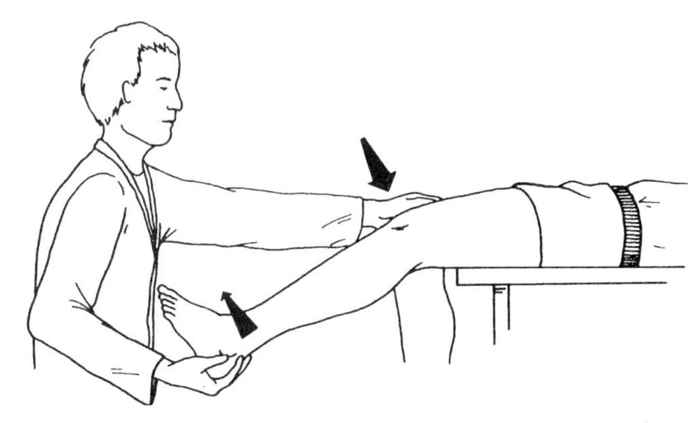

Figure 9. Varus Stress Test. The varus stress test assesses the integrity of the lateral collateral ligament. The patient is placed in the supine position. The examiner places one hand at the medial aspect of the knee joint and the other hand at the heel. The patient's knee is flexed to 30 degrees and varus stress is applied to assess stability of the lateral collateral ligament. The injured knee should be compared to the uninvolved knee.

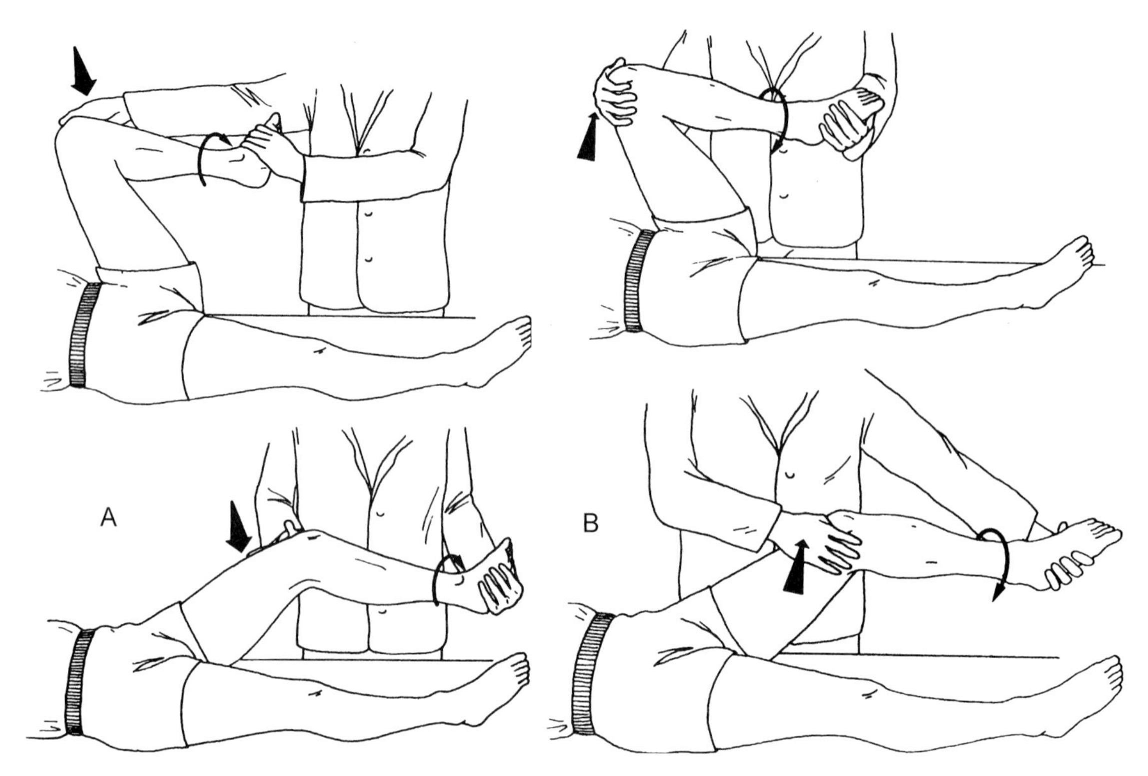

Figure 10. McMurray Test. The patient is placed in the supine position and the knee is placed in full flexion. **(A)** To test the lateral meniscus, a combined external rotation and valgus stress is applied as the knee is extended. **(B)** To test the medial meniscus, the knee again starts in flexion. Combined internal rotation and varus stress are applied as the knee is extended. A meniscal tear is suspected when either pain or a palpable click is elicited with these maneuvers.

Table 1

Common Causes of Knee Pain by Age Group and Location

Location	Children and Adolescents	Adults	Older Adults
Medial	Osteochondritis desiccans	Medial collateral ligament sprain Medial meniscal tear Medial plica syndrome Pes anserine bursitis	Osteoarthritis
Lateral		Iliotibial band syndrome Lateral collateral ligament sprain Lateral meniscal tear	Osteoarthritis
Anterior	Osgood-Schlatter disease Patellar subluxation Patellar tendonitis	Patellofemoral pain syndrome	Osteoarthritis
Posterior		Baker cyst	Baker cyst
Diffuse	Osteochondritis desiccans	Inflammatory conditions Septic arthritis ACL or PCL injury	Osteoarthritis Gout and pseudogout

ACL, anterior cruciate ligament; PCL, posterior cruciate ligament with twisting motions, or with blows to the lateral aspect of the knee. The patient frequently reports hearing or feeling a popping sensation at the time of the injury and has pain that prohibits further activity. If swelling occurs within 2 hours of the injury, rupture of the ligament and hemarthrosis is likely. If hemarthrosis is not present by 24 hours, an ACL tear is unlikely.

Examination: Examination reveals a moderate to severe joint effusion that limits range of motion. The anterior drawer test or Lachman test is positive, though swelling can cause a false-negative test. Radiographs are indicated to rule out tibial spine avulsion fracture.

Treatment: The patient suspected of having an ACL rupture should be referred to an orthopedist for further management.

Crystal-Induced Arthropathies (Gout and Pseudogout)

Presentation: Acute pain and swelling of the knee in the absence of trauma should suggest the possibility of gout or pseudogout (infection also should be considered). In addition to the first metatarsal phalangeal joint, the knee is commonly affected in gout and pseudogout.

Examination: Examination reveals warmth, swelling, erythema, and tenderness. Slight movements of the knee joint cause significant pain. Arthrocentesis is necessary for definitive diagnosis. Polarized-light microscopy of the synovial fluid reveals negatively birefringent rods in gout and positively birefringent rhomboid crystals in pseudogout.

Treatment: Elevation, limited weight-bearing, and nonsteroidal anti-inflammatory drugs (NSAIDs) are the standard therapy for an acute attack of gout or pseudogout.

Iliotibial Band Tendonitis

Presentation: Iliotibial band (IT) tendonitis is an overuse injury common in runners and cyclists caused by friction between the iliotibial band and the lateral femoral condyle. Patients complain of pain at the lateral aspect of the knee, which is aggravated by activities such as climbing stairs and running downhill.

Examination: Examination reveals tenderness at the lateral epicondyle of the femur approximately 3 cm above the joint line.

Treatment: Crepitus may be present. Iliotibial band tendonitis is treated with stretching of the IT band, reducing offending activities, ice, NSAIDs, and sometimes with steroid injection.

Infection

Presentation: Infection of the knee joint may occur in patients of any age, but occurs more often in patients with insufficient immune systems. The patient typically reports acute onset of pain and swelling without preceding trauma.

Examination: Examination reveals warmth, swelling, significant tenderness, and pain with even slight movement of the knee.

Treatment: Fever and chills may be present. Arthrocentesis, Gram stain, and culture are required. Treatment is with intravenous antibiotics, but may require surgical intervention.

Lateral Collateral Ligament Sprain

Presentation: Lateral collateral ligament sprain is caused by varus stress to the knee such as planting the foot and turning toward the same knee. The patient reports immediate onset of pain.

Examination: Examination reveals point tenderness at the lateral joint line over the lateral collateral ligament. Varus stress testing produces pain with sprains and instability with complete rupture of the ligament.

Treatment: Sprains are treated with immobilization in a splint, ice, and compression. Activities may be resumed and muscle strengthening started as improvement occurs. Suspected ligament rupture should be treated with splinting and orthopedic evaluation.

Medial Collateral Ligament Sprain

Presentation: MCL sprains are relatively uncommon and typically are due to valgus stress on the knee, such as a blow to the lateral aspect of the knee. The patient reports immediate pain and swelling at the medial aspect of the knee.

Examination: Examination reveals point tenderness at the medial joint line. Valgus stress testing reproduces the pain. Instability of the joint with valgus stress testing indicates rupture of the ligament.

Treatment: Sprains are treated with immobilization in a splint, ice, and compression. Activities may be resumed and muscle strengthening started as improvement occurs. Suspected ligament rupture should be treated with splinting and orthopedic evaluation.

Medial Plica Syndrome

Presentation: The plica is a redundancy of the joint synovium, which is found at the medial aspect of the knee. This plica can become inflamed with overuse. The patient typically presents with acute medial knee pain after an increase in physical activities.

Examination: Examination reveals a thickened band medial to the patella. No effusion is present, and the remainder of the knee exam is unremarkable.

Treatment: Treatment is with arthroscopic surgical release.

Meniscal Tear

Presentation: Meniscal tear typically occurs with twisting motions of the knee while the foot is planted. The patient reports acute onset of pain followed by swelling several hours later. Meniscal tear also can occur with a prolonged degenerative process such as with chronic ACL instability. The patient with a meniscal tear usually reports recurrent knee pain and swelling. The patient usually reports episodes of catching or locking of the knee, and may report that the knee recurrently collapses.

Examination: Examination reveals tenderness along the medial or lateral joint line, and an effusion may be present. Pain may be elicited with complete flexion. The McMurray test may be positive, but a negative test does not rule out a meniscal tear.

Treatment: For acute tears, the knee should be immobilized for several weeks, along with ice and analgesics. Meniscal tears sometimes heal over a period of approximately 6 weeks, during which time quadriceps strengthening exercises should be employed. A meniscal tear that does not heal should be evaluated by an orthopedist. An acute injury associated with inability to reach complete extension should be seen within 24 hours. Severe tears associated with collapsing, as well as those in which ligamentous tears cannot be excluded should be referred to an orthopedist.

Osteoarthritis

Presentation: Osteoarthritis, also known as degenerative arthritis, typically occurs in older patients and presents with knee pain that is worsened by weight-bearing activities and improved by rest. The patient often reports morning stiffness that gradually improves with activity.

Examination: Examination may reveal tenderness along the medial joint line, lateral joint line, or along the borders of the patella with a positive patellar compression test. An effusion may be present, there may be loss of muscle tone around the knee, and crepitus may be present with range of motion. When osteoarthritis is suspected, weight-bearing radiographs should be obtained. In early disease, radiographs may be normal but with more advanced disease, radiographs reveal joint-space narrowing, osteophyte formation, subchondral sclerosis, and cystic changes.

Treatment: Treatment consists of enough activity to maintain strength and flexibility but not so much as to cause further inflammation. Acetaminophen and NSAIDs are helpful. Glucosamine with chondroitin may provide symptomatic improvement over time. Heat may be used to relieve stiffness and ice can be used when the knee is inflamed. Quadriceps strengthening is helpful, and weight loss should be encouraged in the overweight patient. Injection of the knee with cortisone may be performed during exacerbations of inflammation. Joint replacement may be necessary in advanced disease.

Patellar Tendonitis

Presentation: Patellar tendonitis, also known as jumper's knee, is an inflammation of the patellar tendon most frequently occurring in teenage boys. Patients typically complain of long-standing anterior knee pain that is worsened by activities such as running.

Examination: Examination reveals tenderness over the patellar tendon.

Treatment: Patellar tendonitis is treated with rest (decreasing or eliminating the offending activity), NSAIDs, ice, and compression. Injection with cortisone is contraindicated due to the risk of tendon rupture.

Patellar Subluxation

Presentation: Patellar subluxation typically presents with the complaint of anterior knee pain and a sensation of the knee intermittently giving way. It most commonly occurs in girls and young women.

Examination: Examination reveals peripatellar tenderness, a positive patellar apprehension test, and a patellar that tracks laterally. A mild effusion usually is present.

Treatment: Treatment consists of quadriceps strengthening exercises, which may be conducted under the supervision of a physical therapist. A patellar brace may be helpful. In refractory cases, surgery may be necessary.

Patellofemoral Pain Syndrome (Chondromalacia)

Presentation: Patellofemoral pain syndrome is a common condition in which the patient usually complains of a vague aching in the anterior knee, most often occurring after periods of prolonged sitting. Squatting, kneeling, or walking up or down stairs also may exacerbate the pain. This condition occurs more often in females, teenagers, young adults, and runners.

Examination: Examination reveals patellar crepitus with range of motion, a positive patellar compression test, and sometimes a mild effusion.

Treatment: Treatment is with modification of activities, NSAIDs, and quadriceps strengthening exercises. A patellar brace may be helpful.

Pes Anserine Bursitis

Presentation: The pes anserine bursa is formed by the insertion of the sartorius, gracilis, and semitendinosus muscles at the anteromedial aspect of the proximal tibia. Overuse can cause the bursa to become inflamed. The patient complains of pain at the medial aspect of the knee that is worsened with repetitive flexion and extension.

Examination: Examination reveals tenderness at the insertion of the anserine tendon. Valgus stress testing may reproduce the pain.

Treatment: Treatment is with rest, ice, and NSAIDs. Steroid injection frequently improves symptoms.

Popliteal Cyst (Baker Cyst)

Presentation: A Baker cyst typically presents as a painless or mild to moderately painful swelling in the popliteal space.

Examination: Examination reveals a cystic fullness at the medial aspect of the popliteal fossa. A Baker cyst may be a bursa associated with the semimembranosus or gastrocnemius muscles, or it may be associated with intra-articular knee problems.

Treatment: Therapy for a Baker cyst is focused on treating the underlying knee problem if a problem is suspected. Surgical excision is seldom indicated.

Posterior Cruciate Ligament Injury

Presentation: PCL injury is rare, and typically occurs when significant force is applied to the tibia while the knee is flexed, as when the knee strikes the dashboard in a motor vehicle accident.

Examination: The posterior drawer test may be positive.

Treatment: The patient with suspected PCL injury should be referred to an orthopedist for further management.

Tibial Apophysitis (Osgood-Schlatter Disease)

Presentation: Tibial apophysitis is a relatively common cause of knee pain, particularly in teenage boys involved in athletics. Patients complain of anterior knee pain that waxes and wanes in intensity over a period of weeks to months. The pain typically worsens with certain activities such as walking up and down stairs, squatting, and jumping.

Examination: Examination reveals tenderness, often with a palpable lump, over the tibial tubercle. The pain may be reproduced with resisted active extension of the knee. Radiographs may or may not show fragmentation at the tubercle.

Treatment: Tibial apophysitis is treated by decreasing the offending activity, NSAIDs, and ice. The condition disappears when the apophysis closes.

Osteochondritis Desiccans

Presentation: In osteochondritis desiccans, a piece of articular cartilage becomes necrotic for unknown reasons and can break off the femoral surface with or without a piece of attached bone. The medial femoral condyle is most commonly affected, and this condition is usually found in teenagers and young adults. The piece of cartilage becomes a loose body in the joint causing vague, poorly localized knee pain along with recurrent effusion and morning stiffness. Symptoms of locking or catching may be reported.

Examination: Tenderness may be found under the patella or along the medial femoral condyle. An effusion may be present. Radiographs may reveal the osteochondral lesion at the medial femoral condyle or a loose body in the joint. Arthroscopy may be necessary to make the diagnosis.

Treatment: If osteochondritis desiccans is suspected, the patient should be referred to an orthopedist for definitive diagnosis and management.

REFERENCES

Bergfeld J, Ireland ML, Wojtys EM, Glaser V. Pinpointing the cause of acute knee pain. Patient Care 1997;31(18):100–107.

Birnbaum JS. The Musculoskeletal Manual, 2nd ed. Philadelphia, WB Saunders, 1986, pp 167–200.

Brandt KD. Management of osteoarthritis. In: Kelley WN, ed. Textbook of Rheumatology, 5th ed. Philadelphia, WB Saunders, 1997, pp 1394–1403.

Calmbach WL, Hutchens M. Evaluation of patients presenting with knee pain: Part I. History, physical examination, radiographs, and laboratory tests. Am Fam Physician 2003;68:907–912.

Calmbach WL, Hutchens M. Evaluation of patients presenting with knee pain: Part II. Differential diagnosis. Am Fam Physician 2003;68:917–922.

Cox JS, Blanda JB. Peripatellar pathologies. In: DeLee J, Drez D, Stanitski CL, eds. Orthopaedic Sports Medicine: Principles and Practice, vol 3. Pediatric and Adolescent Sports Medicine. Philadelphia, WB Saunders, 1994, pp 1249–1260.

DeLee JC, Drez D Jr. DeLee and Drez's Orthopaedic Sports Medicine: Principles and Practice, 2nd ed. Philadelphia, WB Saunders, 2003.

Dunn JF. Osgood-Schlatter disease. Am Fam Physician 1990;41:173–176.

Kelley WN, Wortmann RL. Crystal-associated synovitis. In: Kelley WN, ed. Textbook of Rheumatology, 5th ed. Philadelphia, WB Saunders, 1997, pp 1313–1351.

Magee DJ. Knee. Orthopedic Physical Assessment, 4th ed. Philadelphia, WB Saunders, 2002, pp 661–763.

McCune WJ, Golbus J. Monoarticular arthritis. In: Kelley WN, ed. Textbook of Rheumatology, 5th ed. Philadelphia, WB Saunders, 1997, pp 371–380.

McMurray TP. The semilunar cartilage. Br J Surg 1942;29:407–414.

Micheli LF, Foster TE. Acute knee injuries in the immature athlete. Instr Course Lect 1993;42: 473–480.

Reginato AJ, Reginato AM. Diseases associated with deposition of calcium pyrophosphate or hydroxyapatite. In: Kelley WN, ed. Textbook of Rheumatology, 5th ed. Philadelphia, WB Saunders, 1997, pp 1352–1367.

Ruffin MT 5th, Kiningham RB. Anterior knee pain; the challenge of patellofemoral syndrome. Am Fam Physician 1993;47:185–194.

Schenck RC Jr, Goodnight JM. Osteochondritis dissecans. J Bone Joint Surg [Am] 1996;78:439–456.

Smith BW, Green GA. Acute knee injuries: Part I. History and physical examination. Am Fam Physician 1995;51:615–621.

Stanitski CL. Anterior knee pain syndromes in the adolescent. Instr Course Lect 1994;43:211–220.

Tandeter HB, Shvartzman P, Stevens MA. Acute knee injuries: Use of decision rules for selective radiograph ordering. Am Fam Physician 1999;60: 2599–2608.

Walsh WM. Knee injuries. In: Mellion MB, Walsh WM, Shelton GL, eds. The Team Physician's Handbook, 2nd ed. St. Louis, Mosby, 1997, pp 554–578.

“I Can’t Paint Anymore”

Examinee Prompt

You are seeing this 38-year-old man in your office for a chief complaint of "shoulder pain." Please complete the following tasks:

- ❑ Obtain a focused history relevant to this patient's complaint.
- ❑ Perform an appropriate physical examination.
- ❑ Outline a course of treatment for the patient, as well as follow-up, if necessary.

You have 15 minutes to complete your visit with the patient. When you have all of the information that you will need, you may leave the examination room. Following your visit with the patient, you will be asked to generate a differential diagnosis as well as a treatment plan. In this station, you will be asked to write a complete progress note using the standard SOAP (Subjective, Objective, Assessment and Plan) format. You will have 10 additional minutes to complete the progress note.

Patient Prompt

Background: You are a 38-year-old house painter who has had 6 weeks of right shoulder pain.

Chief Complaint: Right shoulder pain

History of the Present Illness: 38-year-old right-hand dominant man who complains of 6 weeks of right shoulder pain. The pain seemed to develop gradually but now is quite uncomfortable. You work as a house painter and are finding it difficult to make it through an entire day of work because of the pain. The pain seems to be worse when working with the arms over the head. The pain also makes it uncomfortable to sleep. There is no history of trauma to the shoulder, shoulder problems, or shoulder surgery.

Past Medical History: Unremarkable

Past Surgical History: Open reduction and internal fixation of the right femur 9 years ago as the result of a motor vehicle accident.

Medications: Acetaminophen has been tried without significant relief of the pain.

Allergies: No known drug allergies

Family History: All family members are healthy

Social History:

- Works full-time as a house painter
- Married for 12 years with 2 children
- No tobacco use, drinks 3 beers per week
- No travel or pets

Review of Systems: Unremarkable except as outlined in the history of the present illness. No fever, no other joint pains, no muscle weakness, no paresthesias.

Additional Information: Please study the examination sections of this chapter before acting as the standardized patient. You should understand the examination of the knee well in order to tell the examiner what portions of the examination cause you pain.

During the examination, the following are pertinent positives:

- There is no significant abnormality upon visualization. As the examiner visualizes the shoulder, please state that there is no visible abnormality.
- Palpation of the lateral shoulder over the subacromial bursa causes pain.
- Range of motion testing produces pain as the arm is abducted between 60 and 105 degrees. All other range of motion is possible but produces mild discomfort.
- Provocative testing of the rotator cuff causes mild discomfort, but there is no weakness. Please state this if the examiner performs provocative testing of the rotator cuff.
- Neer impingement sign is positive.
- The drop arm test is normal.
- Yergason test for biceps tendonitis is negative.
- The cross arm test is negative.
- The apprehension sign and sulcus test are negative.
- Examination of the neck is unremarkable and Spurling test is negative.

Scoring Sheet

Subjective

- ❑ Occupation and sports activities
- ❑ Onset/duration of pain
- ❑ Location of pain
- ❑ Severity of pain
- ❑ Quality of pain
- ❑ History of trauma to the shoulder
- ❑ Stiffness or loss of range of motion
- ❑ Exacerbating and alleviating factors
- ❑ Swelling
- ❑ Clicking or locking
- ❑ Sensation of instability or joint laxity
- ❑ Previous shoulder problems or shoulder surgery
- ❑ Neck pain

Objective

- ❑ Visual inspection of the shoulder
- ❑ Palpation of at least four structures of the shoulder (e.g., biceps tendon, humerus, anterior glenohumeral joint)
- ❑ Evaluation of distal neurovascular status
- ❑ Range of motion testing, including Apley scratch test
- ❑ Yergason test for biceps tendonitis
- ❑ Provocative testing of the rotator cuff
- ❑ Drop arm test
- ❑ Examination of the neck, including Spurling test

Assessment

- ❑ Rotator cuff tendonitis or impingement syndrome
- ❑ Bonus point for subacromial bursitis

Plan (Credit for up to two of the following items)

- ❑ X-rays of the shoulder
- ❑ Diagnostic injection of the shoulder joint
- ❑ Physical therapy
- ❑ Rest and limitation of work activities
- ❑ Return if symptoms do not improve in the next few weeks

Total Score: _____ / 24

Passing score for this station is 16 items.

Communication and Interpersonal Skills (CIS) Scoresheet

Please rate each of the following items on a scale from 1–10.
These items may be completed by either the standardized patient or another student.

Scoresheet 1

	Poor		Fair		Good		Very Good		Excellent	
Professional appearance	1	2	3	4	5	6	7	8	9	10
Introduces self and shakes hands	1	2	3	4	5	6	7	8	9	10
Nonverbal communication (eye contact, facial expressiveness, body language)	1	2	3	4	5	6	7	8	9	10
Communicates effectively (open-ended questions, avoids jargon)	1	2	3	4	5	6	7	8	9	10
Establishes rapport with patient (empathy, appears nonjudgmental)	1	2	3	4	5	6	7	8	9	10
Allows patient to speak without being interrupted	1	2	3	4	5	6	7	8	9	10
Listens and seems to understand patient's concerns	1	2	3	4	5	6	7	8	9	10
Overall professionalism	1	2	3	4	5	6	7	8	9	10

Total Score:

Passing score for CIS section is 56 points.

Spoken English Proficiency (SEP) Scoresheet

Please rate each of the following items on a scale from 1–10.
These items may be completed by either the standardized patient or another student.

Scoresheet 2

	Poor		Fair		Good		Very Good		Excellent	
Examiner is articulate and easily understood	1	2	3	4	5	6	7	8	9	10
Pronunciation (words pronounced correctly; accent does not hinder communication)	1	2	3	4	5	6	7	8	9	10
Word choice is appropriate	1	2	3	4	5	6	7	8	9	10
Ability to communicate without excessive listener effort required to understand questions or responses	1	2	3	4	5	6	7	8	9	10
Patient's ability to understand the examiner	1	2	3	4	5	6	7	8	9	10
Examiner's ability to understand the patient	1	2	3	4	5	6	7	8	9	10

Total Score:

Passing score for SEP section is 42 points.

Approach to the Patient with Shoulder Pain

Anatomy Overview

The humerus, glenoid, scapula, acromion, and clavicle make up the bony structures of the shoulder. The glenohumeral joint capsule consists of a fibrous capsule, ligaments, and the glenoid labrum. The rotator cuff muscles (supraspinatus, infraspinatus, teres minor, and subscapularis) and the scapular rotators (trapezius, serratus anterior, rhomboids, and levator scapulae) provide dynamic stability for the shoulder. The deltoid and latissimus dorsi also assist in movement of the shoulder (Figure 1).

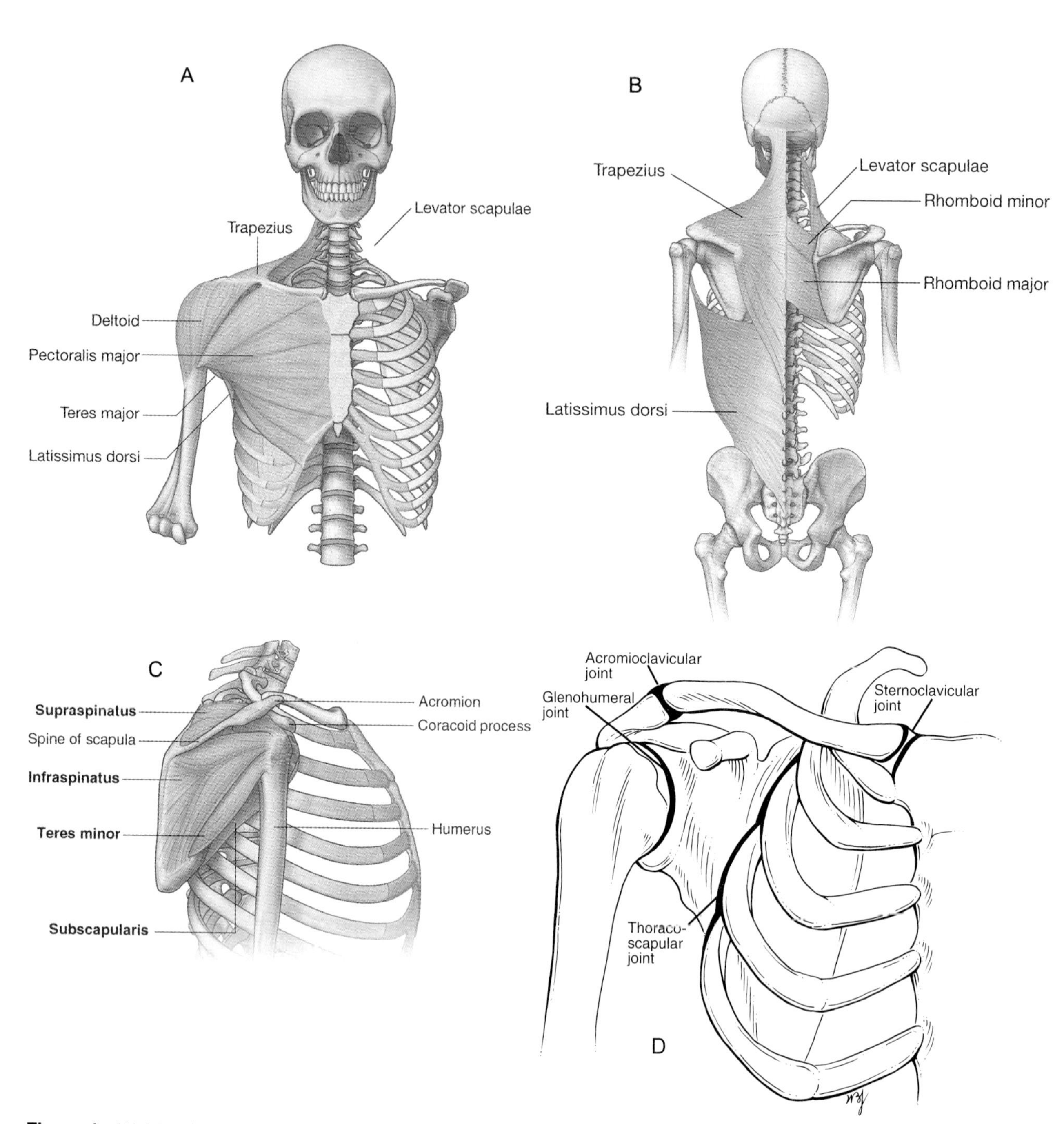

Figure 1. **(A)** Muscles of the anterior shoulder. **(B)** Muscles of the posterior shoulder. **(C)** Rotator cuff muscles. **(D)** Bony anatomy of shoulder, anterior view.

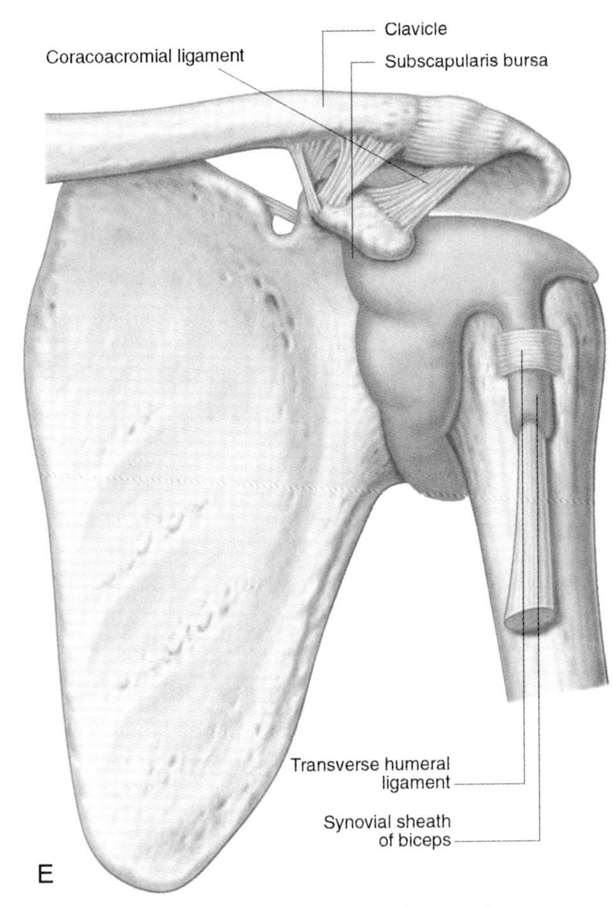

Figure 1. (Cont'd) (E) Deeper view of the anterior aspect of shoulder.

History

The following historical items should be obtained from any patient presenting with a complaint of acute or chronic shoulder pain:

- Age of patient
- Dominant hand
- Occupation and sports activities
- Chronicity of pain
- Quality of pain
- Relieving and exacerbating factors (such as throwing a ball)
- Impact of the pain on work and other daily activities
- Stiffness or loss of range of motion
- Locking
- Catching
- Swelling
- Radiation of pain
- Any sensation of joint laxity
- History of trauma
- Prior shoulder problems or shoulder surgery
- Neck pain
- Muscle weakness or paresthesias
- Other joint pains
- When indicated, historical questions that may elicit a cardiac, pulmonary, gastric, or metastatic cause of the patient's shoulder pain.

Examination

A complete examination of the shoulder includes each of the following items, which are discussed in detail below:

- Inspection of the shoulder
- Palpation of the major structures of the shoulder
- Assessment of the distal neurovascular status, especially in cases of trauma
- Range of motion testing (Figure 2)
- Yergason test for biceps tendonitis (Figure 3)
- Evaluation of the rotator cuff (Figures 4–6)
- Apley scratch test (Figure 7)
- Neer impingement sign (Figure 8)
- Drop arm test (Figure 9)
- Cross arm test (Figure 10)
- Apprehension test (Figure 11)
- Sulcus sign for inferior glenohumeral instability (Figure 12)
- Examination of the neck and Spurling test (Figure 13)

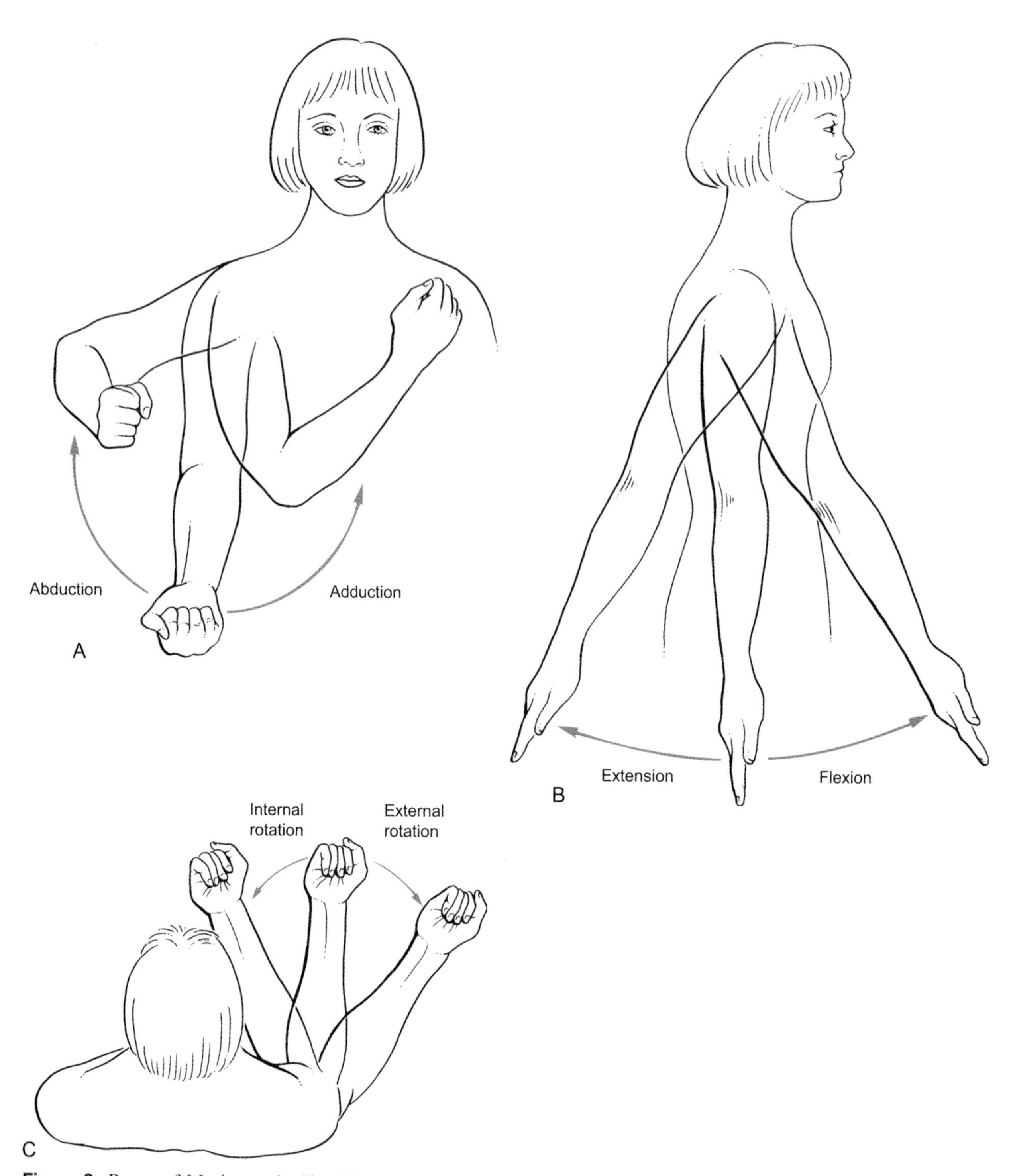

Figure 2. Range of Motion at the Shoulder. **(A)** Abduction and adduction. **(B)** Flexion and extension. **(C)** Internal and external rotation.

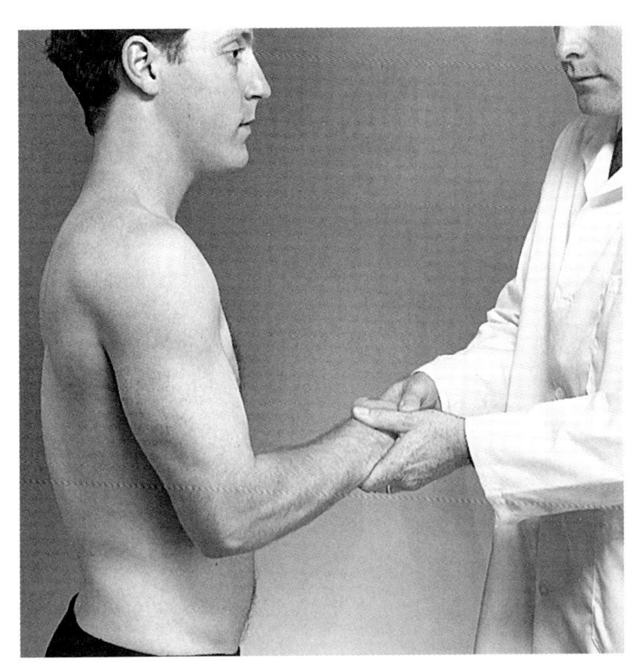

Figure 3. Yergason Test for Biceps Tendonitis. The patient is placed in the seated position and the elbow is flexed to 90 degrees. The patient is asked to supinate the arm and flex the elbow while the examiner grasps the wrist and resists these motions. Pain at the biceps tendon indicates biceps tendonitis.

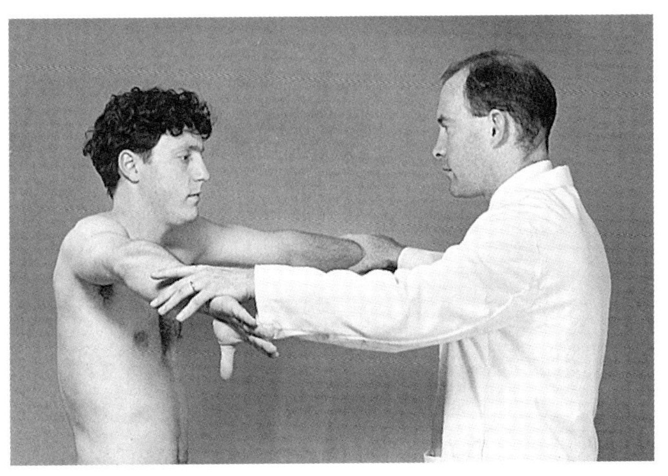

Figure 4. Supraspinatus. The supraspinatus is tested with the "empty can test." The patient is asked to abduct the arms, extend the elbows, and point the thumbs downward. The patient then attempts to elevate the arms against resistance. Pain or weakness may indicate a tear of the supraspinatus.

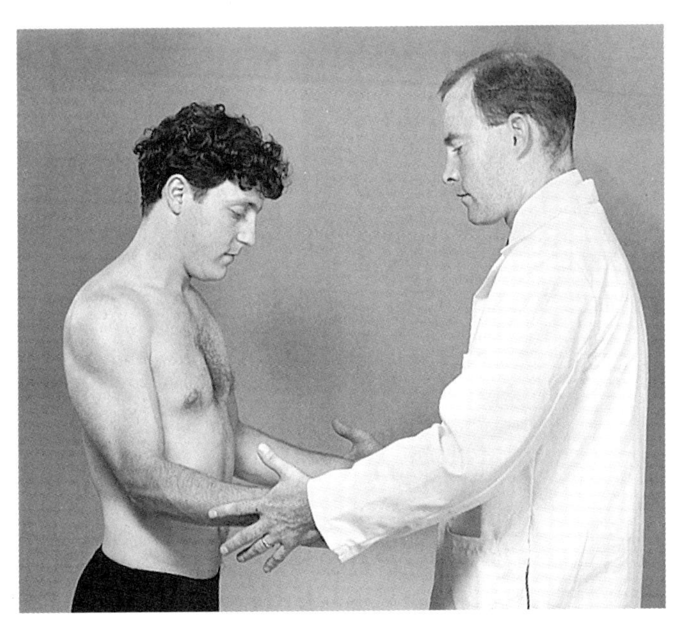

Figure 5. Infraspinatus and Teres Minor. The patient's arms are placed at the sides with the elbows flexed to 90 degrees. The patient attempts to externally rotate the arms against resistance. Pain or weakness may indicate a tear of the infraspinatus or teres minor.

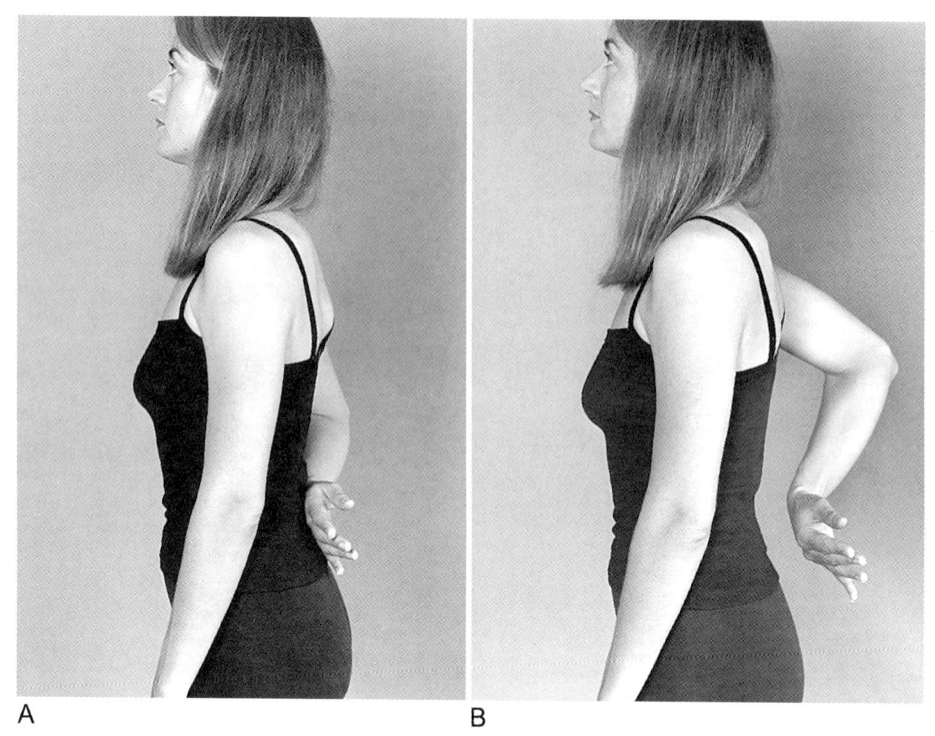

Figure 6. Subscapularis. The patient rests the dorsum of the hand on the back in the lumbar area and is asked to lift the hand off the back, which requires further internal rotation of the arm. Inability to perform this maneuver suggests injury to the subscapularis muscle. Pain or weakness may indicate a tear of the subscapularis.

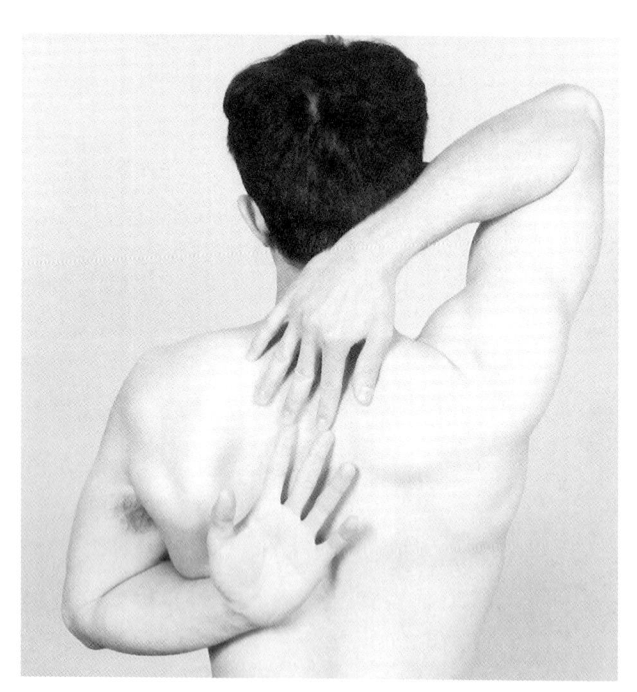

Figure 7. Apley Scratch Test. The Apley scratch test helps assess range of motion in the shoulder. The patient is first asked to reach behind the head and touch the superior aspect of the opposite scapula, which evaluates abduction and external rotation. The patient is then asked to reach behind the back and touch the inferior aspect of the opposite scapula, which evaluates internal rotation and abduction.

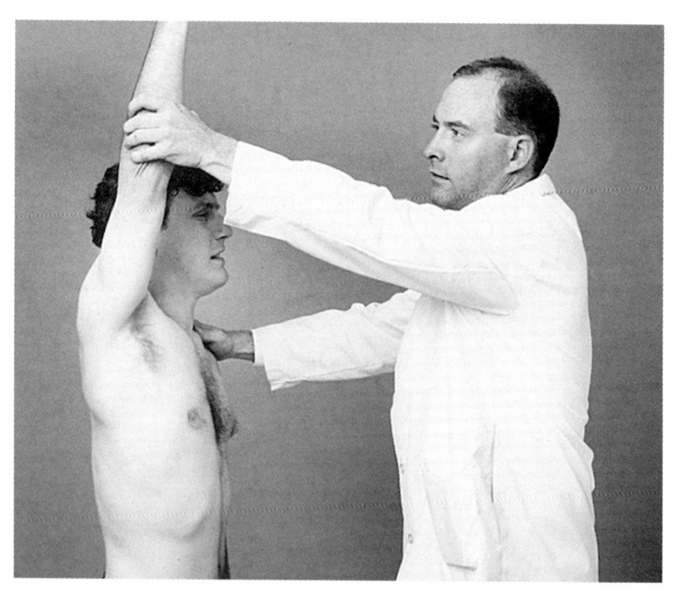

Figure 8. Neer Impingement Sign. The patient's arm is fully pronated and the shoulder is placed in forced flexion while the scapula is stabilized by the examiner. Pain during this maneuver is a sign of subacromial impingement as the rotator cuff tendons are pinched under the coracoacromial arch.

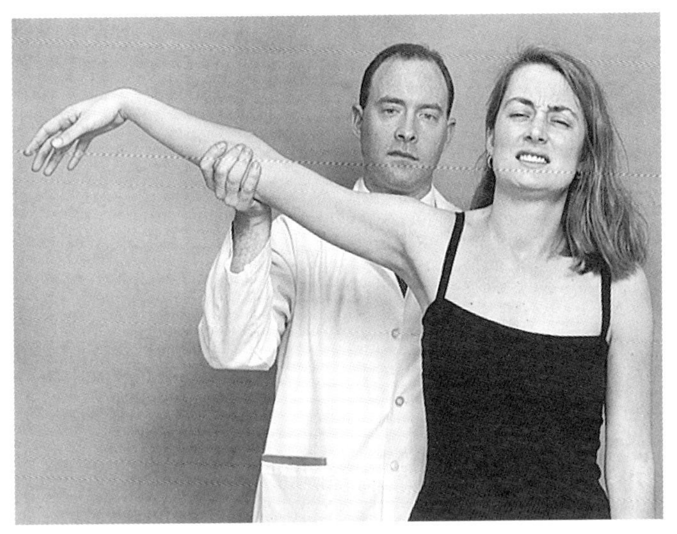

Figure 9. Drop Arm Test. The drop arm tests aids in diagnosis of a possible rotator cuff tear. The patient's arm is passively elevated to 150 degrees, and the patient is asked to slowly lower the arm to the waist. A rotator cuff tear or supraspinatus dysfunction may cause the arm to drop to the patient's side. It should be noted that a patient with a rotator cuff tear may be able to lower the arm slowly to 90 degrees as the deltoid muscle assists in this motion. However, the patient will be unable to continue the maneuver from the 90-degree point down to the waist.

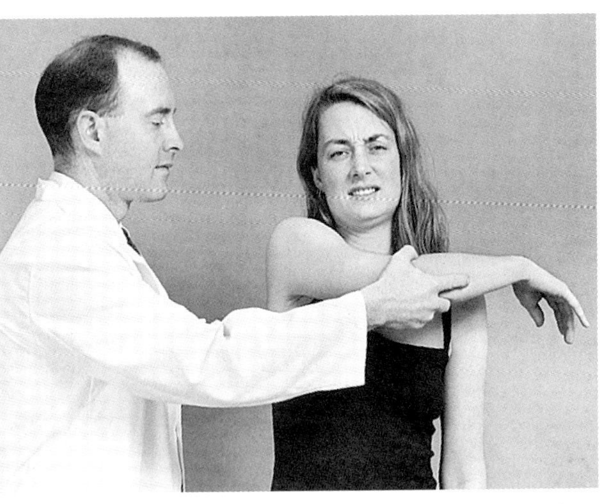

Figure 10. Cross Arm Test. The cross arm test aids in the diagnosis of acromioclavicular joint dysfunction. The patient elevates the affected arm to 90 degrees in front of the body and then adducts the arm across the body. Pain in the area of the acromioclavicular joint suggests dysfunction of this joint.

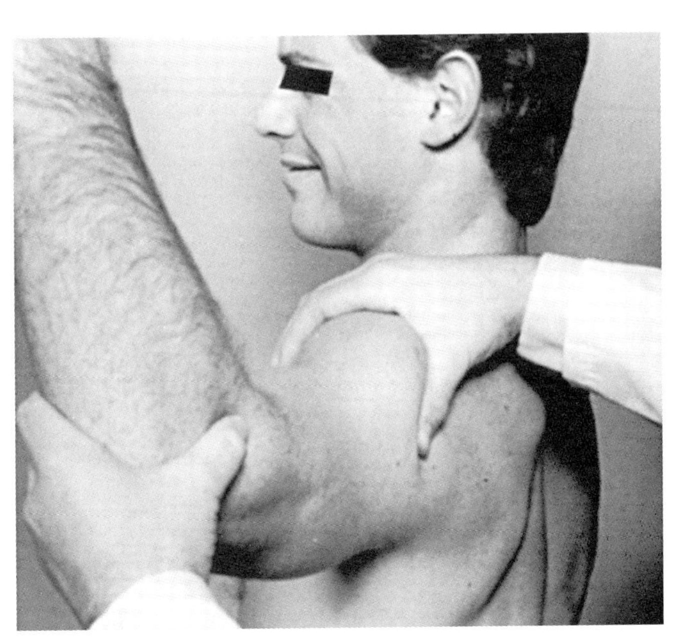

Figure 11. Apprehension Test. The apprehension test assesses for anterior glenohumeral instability. The patient is placed in a seated position and the shoulder is abducted to 90 degrees and the elbow flexed 90 degrees. The examiner externally rotates the arm and applies light anterior pressure to the humerus. Pain or apprehension about the feeling that the shoulder will dislocate represents a positive test, indicating anterior glenohumeral instability.

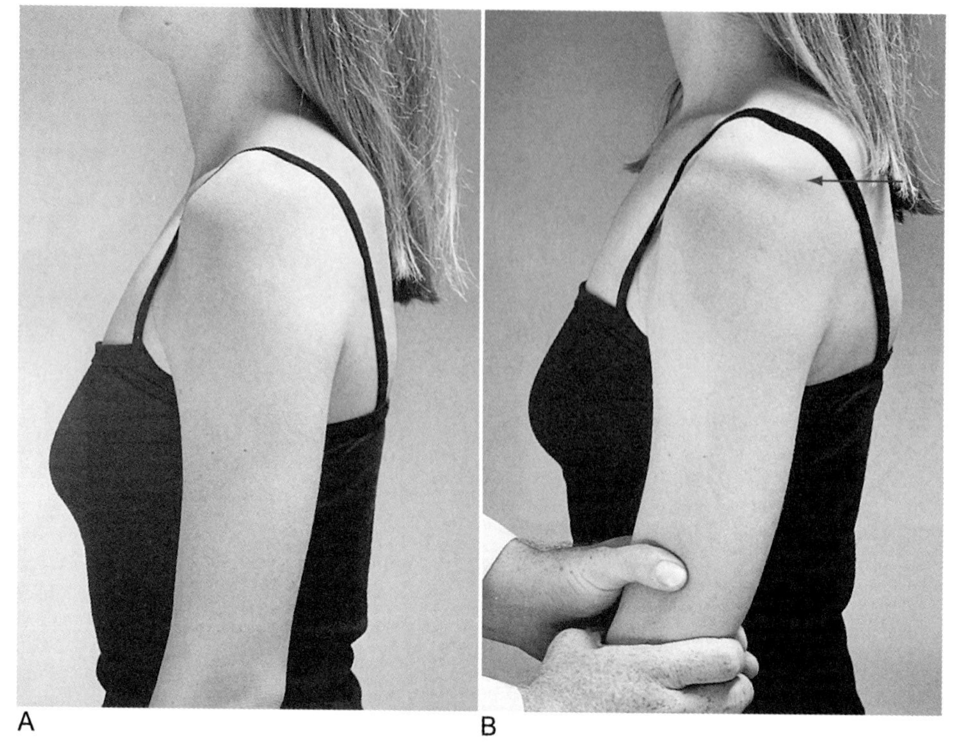

Figure 12. Sulcus Sign. The patient is asked to stand with the arms at the sides. The examiner grasps the elbow and applies downward pressure. The appearance of a sulcus or depression inferior to the acromion indicates that the humerus has migrated inferiorly. The presence of a sulcus suggests inferior glenohumeral instability.

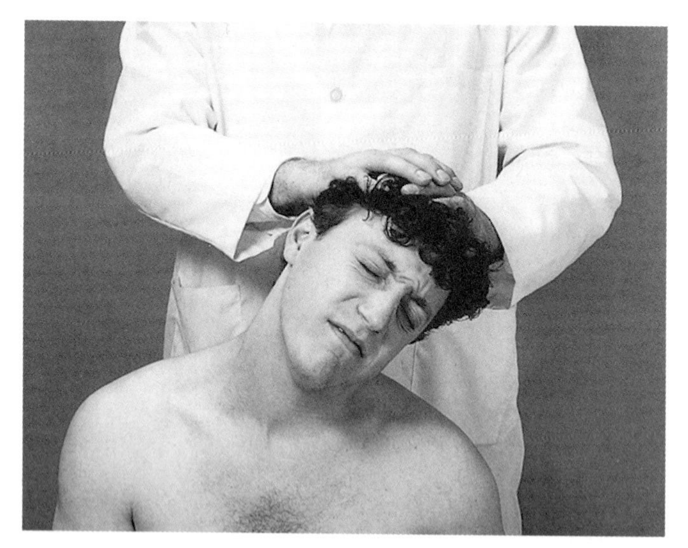

Figure 13. Spurling Test. Spurling test is used to evaluate for cervical root disorders in a patient with shoulder pain that is suspected of having a cervical etiology. The patient is placed in the seated position. The patient's neck is extended and rotated toward the affected shoulder while an axial load is placed on the spine by pressing down on the patient's head. Reproduction of the patient's shoulder pain indicates possible cervical nerve root compression.

Inspection

The patient should be appropriately disrobed to allow proper inspection of both shoulders. The way in which the patient moves and carries the shoulder should be noted. Visual inspection may provide information about swelling, scars, ecchymosis, muscle atrophy, asymmetry, deformity, or scapular winging.

Palpation

The major structures of the shoulder should be palpated for tenderness or deformity. The structures to be palpated include the humerus, acromion, scapula, coracoid process, anterior glenohumeral joint, biceps tendon, acromioclavicular joint, and scapuloclavicular joint. The cervical spine also should be thoroughly palpated.

Range of Motion Testing

Active and passive range of motion should be completely assessed and compared with the unaffected shoulder. A loss of active range of motion with normal passive range of motion suggests muscle weakness rather than true joint pathology. Limitation due to pain of elevation only is suggestive of rotator cuff tendonitis.

Provocative Testing of the Rotator Cuff

When evaluating the rotator cuff, each maneuver should be assessed for weakness and/or pain. A key finding is pain accompanied by weakness, which should be differentiated from weakness that is due to pain.

Specific Causes of Shoulder Pain

Acromioclavicular Joint Sprain (Shoulder Separation)

Presentation: Acromioclavicular (AC) joint sprains and separation usually result from a direct fall onto the shoulder, but may also result from a fall onto an outstretched hand.

Examination: Examination reveals tenderness over the AC joint, and swelling may be present. Radiographs should be performed with a 5- to 10-pound weight in each hand, with comparison made to the unaffected side. AC joint injuries are classified on the basis of six grades of injury. The radiograph is normal in a first-degree sprain but will show increasing degrees of displacement as the grade of injury progresses from 2 through 6.

Treatment: Patients with grade 1 and 2 injuries can be treated with a sling for 1 to 3 weeks until the pain resolves, followed by range of motion exercises. Ice and anti-inflammatory medications should also be used. Grade 3 through 6 injuries should be referred for orthopedic evaluation as operative repair may be necessary (Figure 14).

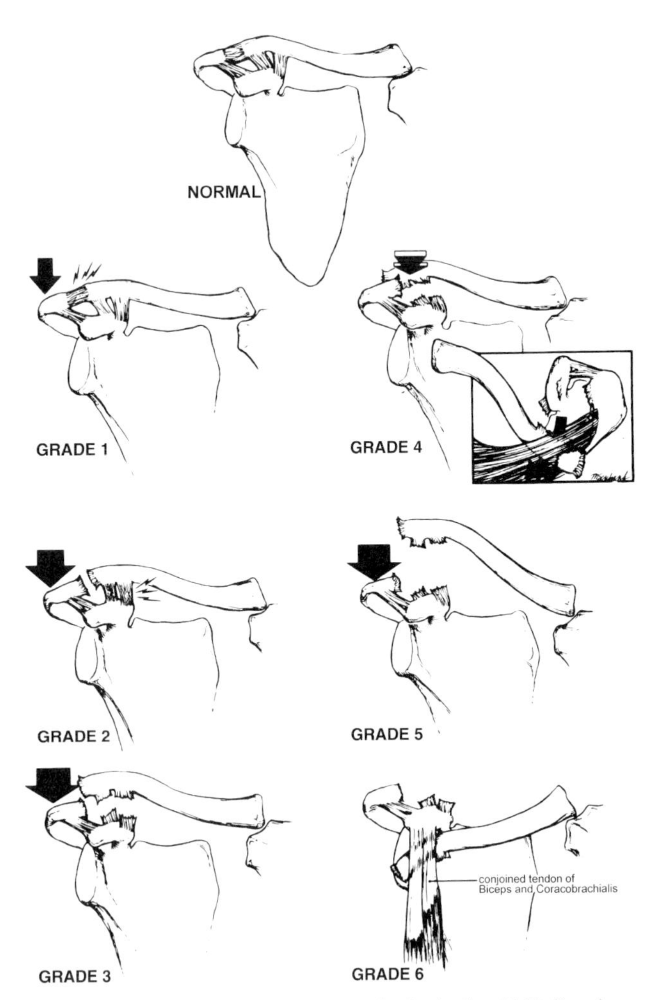

Figure 14. Classification of Acromioclavicular (AC) Sprain. Grade 1: A mild force applied to the shoulder produces strain on the AC ligaments, but the joint remains stable. Grade 2: A force applied to the shoulder disrupts the AC ligaments, but not the coracoclavicular ligaments. Grade 3: A force applied to the shoulder disrupts both the AC and coracoclavicular ligaments. Grade 4: The AC and coracoclavicular ligaments are disrupted, and the distal end of the clavicle is displaced posteriorly. Grade 5: The AC and coracoclavicular ligaments are ruptured and the attachments of the deltoid and trapezius muscles are disrupted, creating a significant separation between the clavicle and the acromion. Grade 6: The AC and coracoclavicular ligaments are disrupted and the distal end of the clavicle is dislocated inferiorly.

Adhesive Capsulitis

Presentation: The patient with adhesive capsulitis typically presents with slowly progressive diffuse pain and limitation of motion of the shoulder in all directions. Adhesive capsulitis often follows another shoulder injury or other recognized cause of shoulder pain. Disuse of the shoulder results in thickening of the joint capsule with restrictive changes in the tissues of the shoulder. The patient often identifies the pain as being near the deltoid insertion and may complain of inability to sleep on the affected shoulder.

Examination: Examination reveals limitation of range of motion in all directions but no significant tenderness to palpation. Radiographs usually are normal, though osteopenia of the humeral head may result due to disuse.

Treatment: Treatment consists of progressive range of motion exercises, often with the assistance of a physical therapist. Anti-inflammatory medications are helpful, and intra-articular steroid injections may speed recovery. The condition improves gradually in a few months, though some residual restriction in range of motion may persist. Failure to improve should raise suspicion for the possibility of an underlying rotator cuff tear.

Biceps Tendonitis

Presentation: Biceps tendonitis usually presents as an overuse injury, most commonly seen in athletes or individuals who perform repetitive, physical work.

Examination: Examination reveals tenderness over the biceps tendon in the area of the bicipital groove. The diagnosis can be confirmed by reproducing the pain with resisted elbow flexion and resisted forearm supination using the Yergason test previously described in this chapter.

Treatment: Treatment consists of rest, ice, and anti-inflammatory medication. In some cases, corticosteroid injection may be helpful, though it does carry a risk of tendon rupture.

Clavicular Fractures

Presentation: Clavicular fractures most commonly occur in the middle one-third of the clavicle, usually as the result of a fall onto an outstretched hand or from a direct blow to the shoulder.

Examination: A gross deformity may be present, and palpation reveals point tenderness. In cases of suspected clavicular fracture, a complete neurovascular examination of the upper extremity should be performed to rule out associated neurologic or vascular injuries. Radiographs should be performed to confirm the diagnosis and identify displaced fractures. Displaced fractures of the proximal or distal clavicle may necessitate orthopedic evaluation.

Treatment: Treatment of most clavicular fractures consists of a sling worn for 2 to 4 weeks. However, this is primarily for patient comfort, and immobilization is not necessary. Repeat radiographs may be obtained in 4 to 6 weeks to ensure proper positioning and healing.

Humerus Fracture

Presentation: Fractures of the proximal humerus are usually caused by a direct blow or a fall onto an outstretched hand. Physical examination reveals point tenderness at the fracture site, and crepitus may be present. Ecchymosis may occur.

Examination: A complete neurovascular examination of the upper extremity is indicated to rule out associated neurologic or vascular injuries. Anteroposterior and lateral radiographs usually will identify the fracture.

Treatment: Treatment of nondisplaced proximal humerus fractures consists of shoulder immobilization. Orthopedic evaluation should be obtained for fractures of the anatomic neck, displaced fractures, fractures associated with neurovascular compromise, and fractures consisting of multiple fracture lines. Repeat radiographs should be obtained in 1 to 2 weeks to ensure that no displacement has occurred.

Labrum Tear

Presentation: Tears of the glenoid labrum typically occur in pitchers and other throwing athletes. These patients complain of a shoulder that clicks or pops with motion.

Examination: Examination reveals clicking or "clunking" as the arm is moved through range of motion, particularly in the overhead position. Signs of laxity may be present, such as a sulcus sign or positive apprehension test. The anterior glenohumeral joint may be tender to palpation. Radiographs usually are normal, and magnetic resonance imaging (MRI) may be required to make the diagnosis.

Treatment: Therapy begins with rest, anti-inflammatory medication, and physical therapy. However, patients who do not respond to this conservative treatment may require surgical repair of the tear.

Osteoarthritis of the Glenohumeral Joint

Presentation: Osteoarthritis of the glenohumeral joint is a relatively uncommon problem that is usually found in older patients or in patients who have had a history of significant shoulder trauma. Osteoarthritis typically causes gradually developing shoulder pain over a period of months to years. The pain is worse after use, and the inflammation may result in loss of passive motion as well as stiffness in the shoulder.

Examination: Examination reveals mild to moderate diffuse tenderness to palpation, pain in all directions of motion, and some limitation in range of motion. Radiographs may reveal a narrowed joint space as well as degenerative changes.

Treatment: Treatment consists of heat, ice, anti-inflammatories, and range of motion exercises. Intra-articular corticosteroid injection may be helpful.

Rotator Cuff Tear

Presentation: Rotator cuff tears are usually degenerative in nature and are most common in older patients following a prolonged syndrome similar to rotator cuff tendonitis. However, rotator cuff tears can also occur in younger patients, usually as the result of trauma. Among athletes, rotator cuff tears are most common among baseball pitchers.

Examination: Examination may reveal a loss of active elevation beyond a certain point. Provocative testing of the rotator cuff, as previously described in this chapter, may reveal weakness of a specific muscle and tendon. Radiographs may reveal calcification of the involved tendon and may reveal migration of the humeral head superiorly.

Treatment: Patients with suspected rotator cuff tear should be sent for orthopedic evaluation. Surgical repair should be considered in younger patients and in selected older patients. Older patients who are not good candidates for surgery can be treated conservatively with rehabilitation.

Rotator Cuff Tendinitis (Impingement Syndrome)

Presentation: Rotator cuff tendonitis typically presents as pain over the anterolateral aspect of the shoulder, often with radiation to the upper arm. A history of overuse is common, and this condition frequently occurs in swimmers, pitchers, and house painters. The pain usually is worse at night and may be aggravated by overhead activities. Patients may complain of a clicking or popping sensation in the affected shoulder.

Rotator cuff tendonitis occurs as the result of impingement of the tendons of the rotator cuff between the bony structures of the coracoacromial arch and the humerus. The impingement occurs with abduction, and usually follows repetitive motions (known as a painful arc).

Examination: Examination reveals pain with elevation of the shoulder, typically between 60 and 105 degrees. Other motions may also be painful. Tenderness may be present over the subacromial bursa because subacromial bursitis may accompany rotator cuff tendonitis. Tenderness may also be present over the biceps tendon as biceps tendonitis may occur in the later stages of impingement.

Radiographs may reveal calcification of the tendon, degenerative changes at the AC joint, and osteophyte formation at the acromion. In uncertain cases, MRI may be needed to help make the diagnosis.

Treatment: Initial treatment is conservative and consists of rest, ice, anti-inflammatory medications, and avoiding overhead activities. Corticosteroid injection may provide significant short-term relief of symptoms. Once the pain has improved, rotator cuff strengthening exercises should be started. Failure to improve may be the result of underlying shoulder instability or a partial rotator cuff tear. Patients who do not respond to therapy should be referred for orthopedic consultation.

Scapular Fracture

Presentation: Scapular fractures are uncommon, and usually are caused by direct trauma to the scapular area.

Examination: Examination reveals tenderness over the fracture site and pain with abduction of the arm. When scapular fracture is suspected, anteroposterior, lateral, and axillary radiographs of the shoulder should be obtained.

Treatment: Treatment consists of the use of a sling for patient comfort. Range of motion exercises should be implemented as soon as the pain improves, preferably within 2 weeks.

Shoulder Dislocation (Subluxation)

Presentation: The humeral head can dislocate anteriorly, posteriorly, or inferiorly in relation to the glenoid fossa, though most shoulder dislocations are anterior. The patient may have a history of previous shoulder dislocation. Shoulder dislocation is especially common in teenagers and young athletes. The characteristic mechanism of injury is indirect trauma in forced abduction and external rotation. Such an injury may occur in falls onto the abducted, externally rotated arm or when a football player attempts to tackle with an outstretched arm.

Examination: The patient typically is in obvious distress, particularly with first-time dislocations. Visual inspection reveals the patient holding the affected arm in external rotation and abduction, often supported by the uninjured arm. The normal rounded contour of the shoulder is lost. Palpation reveals the humeral head to be palpable anteriorly with a dimple in the skin beneath the acromion.

Radiographs should include anteroposterior and lateral views to confirm the diagnosis. A Y-view may be obtained if the anteroposterior position of the humeral head relative to the glenoid fossa is in doubt. Radiographs also may rule out fracture of the humerus or clavicle.

Treatment: Acute dislocation requires reduction. Orthopedic consultation should be obtained for recurrent subluxation.

Shoulder Instability (Recurrent Subluxation)

Presentation: The patient with shoulder instability typically complains of either a sense of instability in the shoulder joint or of a sensation that the shoulder recurrently and painfully goes out of place. The patient with recurrent subluxation almost always has a history of previous shoulder dislocation. Recurrent subluxation is most common in teenagers and young athletes.

Examination: Examination reveals a positive apprehension test, and a positive sulcus sign may be present as well.

Treatment: Though a strengthening program may be helpful, referral for orthopedic consultation usually is necessary for surgical repair.

Subacromial Bursitis

Presentation: The patient with subacromial bursitis usually presents with a complaint of pain over the lateral aspect of the shoulder and usually has a history of recent overuse. Though subacromial bursitis may accompany rotator cuff tendonitis, it may also occur independently.

Examination: Examination reveals tenderness over the lateral shoulder at the location of the subacromial bursa. The lack of a painful arc during abduction differentiates isolated subacromial bursitis from subacromial bursitis accompanying rotator cuff tendonitis. Radiographs are not indicated as this is a clinical diagnosis.

Treatment: Treatment consists of rest and antiinflammatory medications or corticosteroid injection of the bursa.

REFERENCES

Anderson BC. Shoulder. In: Office Orthopedics for Primary Care, Diagnosis and Treatment, 2nd ed. Philadelphia, WB Saunders, 1999, pp 13–47.

Birnbaum JS. In: The Musculoskeletal Manual, 2nd ed. Philadelphia, WB Saunders, 1986, pp 57–71.

Burk DL Jr, Karasick D, Kurtz AB, et al. Rotator cuff tears: Prospective comparison of MR imaging with arthrography, sonography, and surgery. Am J Roentgenol 1989; 153:87–92.

Garrick JG, Webb DR. In: Sports Injuries: Diagnosis and Management, 2nd ed. Philadelphia, WB Saunders, 1999, pp 51–148.

Harryman DT, Sidles JA, Clark JM, et al. Translation of the humeral head on the glenoid with passive glenohumeral motion. J Bone Joint Surg [Am] 1990; 72:1334–1343.

Herzog RJ. Magnetic resonance imaging of the shoulder. J Bone Joint Surg [Am] 1997;79:933–953.

Miniaci A, Salonen D. Rotator cuff evaluation imaging and diagnosis. Orthop Clin North Am 1997; 28:43–58.

Neer CS. Impingement lesions. Clin Orthop 1983; 173:70–77.

Neer CS 2d. Displaced proximal humeral fractures: I. Classification and evaluation. J Bone Joint Surg [Am] 1970;52:1077–1089.

Newberg AH. The radiographic evaluation of shoulder and elbow pain in the athlete. Clin Sports Med 1987; 6:785–809.

Rockwood CA Jr, Williams GR, Young DC. Injuries to the acromioclavicular joint. In: Rockwood CA Jr, Green DP, Bucholz RW, eds. Rockwood and Green's Fractures in Adults. 4th ed. Philadelphia, Lippincott-Raven, 1996, pp 1341–1407.

Woodward TW, Best TM. The painful shoulder: Part I. Clinical evaluation. Am Fam Physician 2000; 61:3079–3088.

Woodward TW, Best TM. The painful shoulder: Part II. Acute and chronic disorders. Am Fam Physician 2000;61:3291–3300.

Yergason RM. Supination sign. J Bone Joint Surg [Am] 1931;13:160.

"My Belly Hurts and I'm Throwing Up"

Examinee Prompt

You are working in an outpatient clinic and are asked to see a 25-year old female patient with a complaint of abdominal pain. Please perform the following tasks:

- ❑ Obtain a focused history relevant to this patient’s chief complaint.
- ❑ Perform an appropriate physical exam
- ❑ Following the examination, write a complete progress note documenting your findings using standard SOAP (Subjective, Objective, Assessment and Plan) format.
- ❑ Provide a differential diagnosis, noting your most likely diagnosis first.
- ❑ Document an initial diagnostic/therapeutic plan.

Please note that some parts of this exam may be deferred. If you would normally examine any body parts but are deferring them with the standardized patient, please include them in your plan on the progress note.

You have 15 minutes to complete your visit with the patient. You will have 10 additional minutes to complete the progress note.

Vital Signs

Temperature .... 101.2°F

Blood pressure 138/86

Heart rate 110

Respiratory rate 16

Patient Prompt

Background: You are seeing this doctor for a complaint of abdominal pain. You are quite worried because until recently you have been in completely good health and are very active.

Chief Complaint: Right-sided abdominal pain

History of the Present Illness: This 25-year-old woman awoke at 3 AM, with vague diffuse abdominal discomfort. The pain was mostly epigastric/periumbilical and constant. The pain was significant enough that it caused difficulty in falling back to sleep. In the morning, breakfast was not eaten due to a lack of appetite. Several hours later, nausea and vomiting developed. The vomit was clear liquid without blood or bile. The pain then migrated to the right lower quadrant. A subjective fever developed, though the patient did not take a temperature. Any movement now causes significant pain, 8/10 in intensity on a pain scale.

Past Medical History: None

Past Surgical History: None

Gynecologic History:
- No pregnancies
- Last menstrual period 2 weeks ago

Medications: None

Allergies: None

Social History:
- Engaged
- Administrative assistant at an illustration company
- Sexually active, monogamous, heterosexual
- Four prior sexual partners
- No tobacco, drugs, or alcohol

Family History: Unknown (adopted)

Review of Systems:
- No upper respiratory infection symptoms
- No recent diarrhea
- No constipation
- Normal bowel movement pattern is every other day
- No blood in stools and no black tarry stools
- No dysuria, frequency, urgency, or hesitancy
- No history of trauma
- No vaginal discharge or pelvic pain

Additional Information: For this station, the examinee is asked to perform a physical examination. You should also respond to the exam appropriately.

A pelvic, genitourinary, and rectal exam will not be performed.

The details of the physical exam are as follows. You should act out the pertinent positives and negatives.

- General appearance: Moderately ill-appearing, nontoxic, appears uncomfortable due to pain.
- Cardiovascular: Unremarkable except mild tachycardia at a rate of 110. Tell the examinee that the heart rate is 110.
- Pulmonary: Unremarkable.
- Abdomen: Flat, rigid abdomen with significant tenderness to palpation in the right lower quadrant. Rebound and guarding are present. Nondistended with normal bowel sounds. Significant pain is present with movement of the body. Positive obturator and psoas signs.
- Back: No right costovertebral angle tenderness.

Abdominal Pain Scoresheet

Subjective

- ❑ Location of pain
- ❑ Onset (rapid vs. gradual)
- ❑ Severity, including use of pain scale
- ❑ Radiation
- ❑ Nature of pain (sharp, colicky, dull, etc.)
- ❑ Nausea/vomiting
- ❑ Anorexia
- ❑ Urinary symptoms (dysuria, hematuria)
- ❑ Diarrhea or constipation
- ❑ Melena or blood in stools
- ❑ Fever or chills
- ❑ Last menstrual period
- ❑ Past medical/surgical history
- ❑ Medications
- ❑ Allergies

Objective

- ❑ Vital signs
- ❑ General appearance: Should indicate some degree of patient discomfort
- ❑ Cardiovascular
- ❑ Lungs: Clear
- ❑ Abdomen (1 point for performing the abdominal exam, and 1 point for each specific point on the progress note: tenderness to palpation in right lower quadrant, rebound and guarding, positive obturator and psoas signs, normal bowel sounds)
- ❑ Back: No costovertebral angle tenderness

Diagnosis

- ❑ Appendicitis (or rule-out appendicitis)

Plan

- ❑ Rectal exam
- ❑ Pelvic exam
- ❑ Complete blood count (CBC)
- ❑ Pregnancy test
- ❑ Urinalysis
- ❑ One of the following: computed tomography (CT) scan of abdomen and pelvis or ultrasound
- ❑ The following should not have been ordered (1 point deducted for each): magnetic resonance imaging (MRI), colonoscopy, upper gastrointestinal (GI)/barium swallow, *Helicobacter pylori* antibody, hepatitis viral serology, stool ova and parasites (O&P), white blood cell count (WBC), culture, pelvic ultrasound (normal), intravenous pyelography (IVP)

Total Score: _____ / 32

Passing score for this station is 22 correct items.

Communication and Interpersonal Skills (CIS) Scoresheet

Please rate each of the following items on a scale from 1–10.
These items may be completed by either the standardized patient or another student.

Scoresheet 1

	Poor		Fair		Good		Very Good		Excellent	
Professional appearance	1	2	3	4	5	6	7	8	9	10
Introduces self and shakes hands	1	2	3	4	5	6	7	8	9	10
Nonverbal communication (eye contact, facial expressiveness, body language)	1	2	3	4	5	6	7	8	9	10
Communicates effectively (open-ended questions, avoids jargon)	1	2	3	4	5	6	7	8	9	10
Establishes rapport with patient (empathy, appears nonjudgmental)	1	2	3	4	5	6	7	8	9	10
Allows patient to speak without being interrupted	1	2	3	4	5	6	7	8	9	10
Listens and seems to understand patient's concerns	1	2	3	4	5	6	7	8	9	10
Overall professionalism	1	2	3	4	5	6	7	8	9	10

Total Score:

Passing score for CIS section is 56 points.

Spoken English Proficiency (SEP) Scoresheet

Please rate each of the following items on a scale from 1–10.
These items may be completed by either the standardized patient or another student.

Scoresheet 2

	Poor		Fair		Good		Very Good		Excellent	
Examiner is articulate and easily understood	1	2	3	4	5	6	7	8	9	10
Pronunciation (words pronounced correctly; accent does not hinder communication)	1	2	3	4	5	6	7	8	9	10
Word choice is appropriate	1	2	3	4	5	6	7	8	9	10
Ability to communicate without excessive listener effort required to understand questions or responses	1	2	3	4	5	6	7	8	9	10
Patient's ability to understand the examiner	1	2	3	4	5	6	7	8	9	10
Examiner's ability to understand the patient	1	2	3	4	5	6	7	8	9	10

Total Score:

Passing score for SEP section is 42 points.

Discussion

A patient who presents with right lower quadrant pain should be considered to have appendicitis until you have convinced yourself otherwise. It is the most common cause of acute abdomen. Though the above presentation is classic, actual cases of acute appendicitis may not be. Your presumptive diagnosis should be made by history and physical exam alone. Labs such as CBC and urinalysis (UA) can be deceiving: a normal CBC is common early in the course. UA may be abnormal as a retrocecal appendix may irritate the ureters. CT scans of the abdomen are gaining more and more use, especially in equivocal cases.

A Systematic Approach to Acute Abdominal Pain

Introduction

A complaint of abdominal pain may present a seemingly overwhelming situation. The broad differential and potential for serious disease can be intimidating unless you have a fundamentally strong understanding of abdominal pain and strategy for dealing with each case. The additional stress of encountering this topic during an exam underscores the importance of having a routine and systematic approach to this clinical scenario. It will soon become very obvious that simply memorizing the extensive differential diagnosis of abdominal pain is in itself inadequate and troublesome.

Key Historical Features

Abdominal Colic: Recognizing a pattern of pain as "colicky" may be instrumental in arriving at a correct diagnosis. Colicky pain tends to be "crampy" in nature and usually waxes and wanes over time. Pain may alternate between severe and stabbing in nature and then subside to a dull ache. Unless there is concurrent peritoneal irritation (see below) the pain may be poorly localized. Colic suggests distention of a hollow viscus as seen in biliary, ureteral, and bowel disease.

Associated Symptoms: The symptoms that accompany abdominal pain may provide important clues to the correct diagnosis. Your familiarity with the review of systems of the various organ systems may be instrumental in helping narrow the differential diagnosis. For example:

- Symptoms made better or worse with meals or with bowel movements suggest a gastrointestinal or biliary tract etiology. Diarrhea, constipation, bright red blood per rectum, or melena also suggests the GI tract as the source of pathology.
- Urinary symptoms such as dysuria, hematuria, frequency, hesitancy, urgency, or nocturia suggest genitourinary pathology.
- Vaginal bleeding or missed menses suggests gynecologic pathology.
- Constitutional symptoms such as fever, anorexia, nausea, and vomiting are much less specific. Their presence or absence do not suggest or rule out any particular disease state.

Radiation of Pain: In specific cases, abdominal pain may radiate to other areas, giving you possible clues to its etiology. For example:

- Pain radiating to the shoulders suggests a subdiaphragmatic process (e.g., hepatitis, splenic abscess, biliary disease).
- Pain radiating to the back may suggest a pancreatic, gastric, aortic, or renal etiology. The ascending and descending colon, both retroperitoneal structures, may cause pain that radiates to the back or flank.
- Pain radiating to the groin or testes may suggest a perirenal process such as a kidney stone or perinephric abscess.

Formulate the Differential Diagnosis Based Upon Cross-Sectional Anatomy

Experienced clinicians often visualize the area of concern and the organ systems in the nearby vicinity. Consider the various diseases of those organs to formulate a differential diagnosis.

For example, right lower quadrant pain may involve the appendix, ovary (cyst), fallopian tube (tubo-ovarian abscess, ectopic pregnancy), colon (diverticulitis), ureter (stone), psoas muscle (abscess), abdominal wall (muscle strain, hernia), or testicle (epididymitis, torsion, orchitis). See Figure 1 for a differential diagnosis of abdominal pain based upon the quadrant involved.

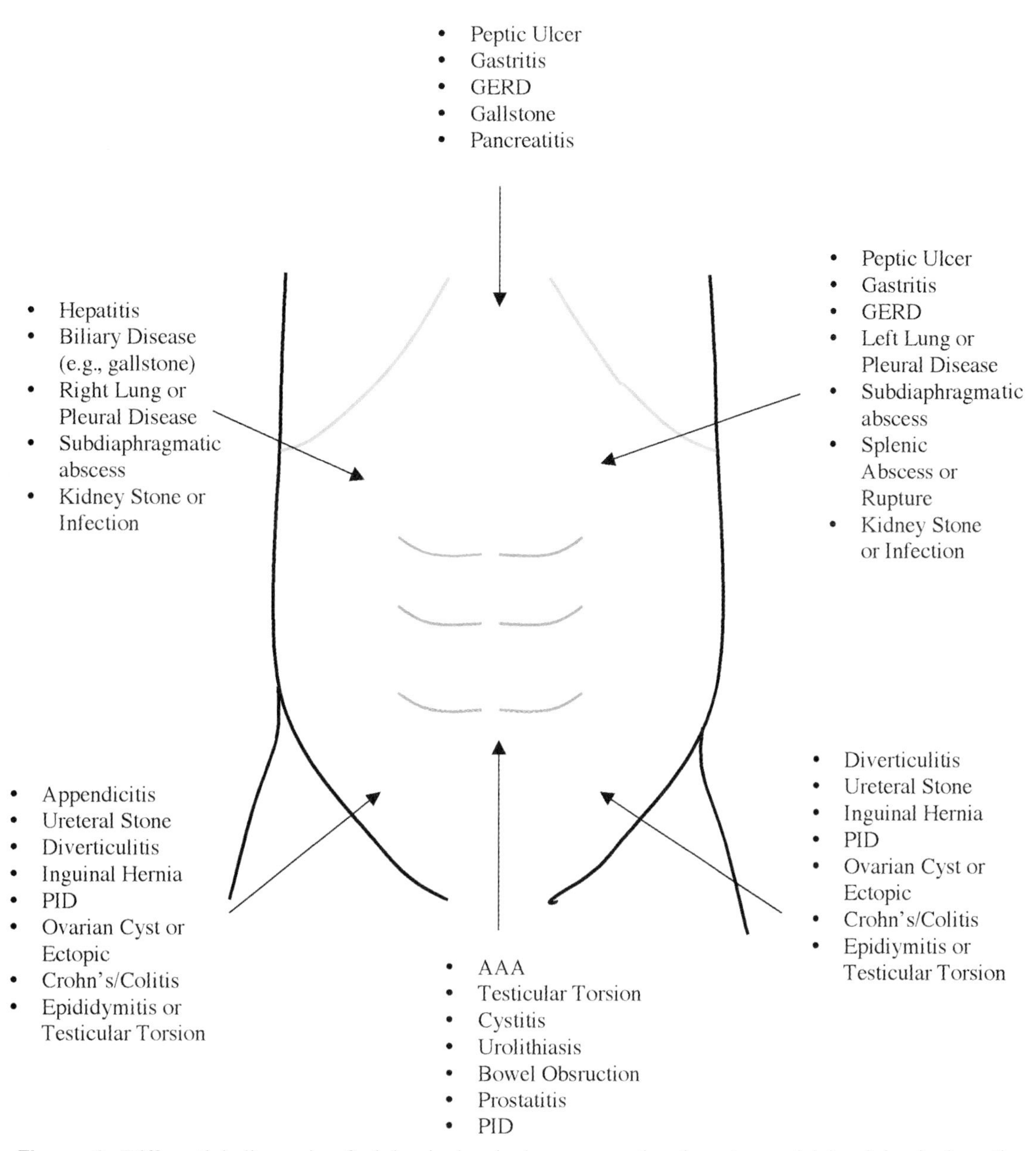

Figure 1. Differential diagnosis of abdominal pain by cross-sectional anatomy. AAA, abdominal aortic aneurysm; GERD, gastroesophageal reflux disease; PID, pelvic inflammatory disease.

Recognize Peritoneal Signs: "The Acute Abdomen"

An integral part of the evaluation of acute abdominal pain is the diagnosis of "the acute abdomen." When an acute abdomen is suspected, surgical evaluation often is necessary.

- Peritoneal signs are those physical exam findings that result from irritation or inflammation of the parietal peritoneum. The patient is often lying very still as any movement exacerbates the pain. Pain is often very well-localized and reproducible with palpation. Guarding or rigidity (involuntary tensing of abdominal muscles), rebound tenderness (pain elicited with the release of deeper palpation), and referred tenderness (percussion or palpation of another area reproduces pain at the site of pathology) are usually present. Other methods of reproducing peritoneal pain include extension at the hip (psoas sign), external rotation of the hip (obturator sign), and shaking the patient's hips. Bowel sounds may be hypoactive or absent.
- Visceral pain should be distinguished from peritoneal pain because it indicates pathology of the abdominal contents without overt peritoneal irritation. This pain is often more

poorly localized, the patient may writhe in pain, and there may be complete absence of focal tenderness to palpation.

Suggested Laboratory and Radiographic Studies in the Workup of Acute Abdominal Pain

Although not all of the following studies are indicated in each case of acute abdominal pain, the studies should be understood well so that they may be ordered appropriately.

- Pregnancy test should be performed for all female patients of reproductive age presenting with abdominal pain.
- CBC provides information about infection and anemia.
- Stool guaiac may diagnose occult GI bleeding.
- UA may provide information about the presence of urinary tract infection or kidney stones.
- Liver function tests (aspartate aminotransferase [AST], alanine aminotransferase [ALT], bilirubin, alkaline phosphatase, and gamma glutamyl transferase [GGT]) may provide information about the presence of hepatic or biliary processes.
- Amylase and lipase may provide data about the presence of pancreatic disease.
- KUB (a plain abdominal radiograph of *k*idney, *u*reters, *b*ladder) may help identify bowel obstruction, perforation, or constipation. A KUB is indicated if significant vomiting is present (especially bilious vomiting) or if small or large bowel obstruction is suspected. It may also be used to screen for radiopaque kidney stones.
- Ultrasound is helpful in identifying gallstones, hydronephrosis, and sometimes appendicitis. However, not all cases of appendicitis are detected, especially in adults.
- CT scan is more expensive than ultrasound but may better visualize some organs. It may be ordered to help identify the cause of acute abdominal pain when an initial ultrasound yields equivocal results. Most cases of abdominal pain resulting from trauma warrant a CT scan. In addition, severe abdominal pain or significant abdominal pain with fever may warrant CT scanning.
- IVP essentially is a KUB with IV contrast dye to image the upper urinary tract. It may help identify kidney stones.
- HIDA scan is a functional test of the gallbladder used for diagnosing acute cholecystitis and acalculous biliary disease. A HIDA scan often can be useful if a screening ultrasound is nondiagnostic in a patient suspected of having biliary disease.
- Upper GI with small bowel follow-through is a study in which the patient swallows oral contrast and fluoroscopic images are taken. This study may identify esophageal, gastric, and small bowel pathology.
- Endoscopy is the examination of the upper and/or lower GI tract using a fiberoptic scope. This study is invasive and requires specialty consultation. It may be helpful in diagnosing mucosal inflammation, polyps, and cancer. Endoscopy may be indicated in the workup of iron-deficiency anemia.

Classic Presentations of Common Diseases

Acute Appendicitis

Presentation: Acute appendicitis commonly begins with anorexia, malaise, nausea/vomiting, and fever. Pain typically begins as diffuse periumbilical discomfort. Later, as the disease progresses, pain becomes localized to the right lower quadrant as peritoneal signs develop.

Examination: UA is usually unremarkable. Elevation of the WBC is common. Radiographs may be normal, or may show a paucity of gas in the right lower quadrant or a calcification called an appendolith. CT scan usually reveals inflammation around the appendix. However, when acute appendicitis is suspected, CT scanning may be unnecessary as the patient may be taken to the operating for surgical exploration.

Treatment: Patients suspected of having acute appendicitis should receive a surgical consultation.

Urolithiasis

Presentation: Urolithiasis, or kidney stones, typically presents with colicky unilateral flank pain with radiation to the ipsilateral groin or testicle as the stone encounters the ureteropelvic junction. Nausea and vomiting are common. Hematuria (gross or microscopic) is common. Fever and leukocytosis are absent unless a concomitant infection is present. As the stone passes distally, it encounters two additional areas of resistance, and pain often migrates. As the ureteral stone traverses the area of the iliac artery, lower abdominal pain develops. Later, when the stone encounters the ureterovesicular junction, suprapubic or groin pain may develop. The KUB may be normal unless the stone is radiopaque (e.g., calcium oxalate).

Examination: A noncontrast abdominal CT is the diagnostic study of choice as it can reveal even radiolucent stones (e.g., uric acid). IVP may show ureteral obstruction or hydronephrosis. Renal ultrasound may also show hydronephrosis.

Treatment: Treatment for smaller stones (<4 mm) is generally symptomatic as these stones usually pass. Adequate analgesia can be provided with nonsteroidal anti-inflammatory drugs (NSAIDs) and narcotic analgesics (such as IV ketorolac with IV morphine or oral hydrocodone, oxycodone, hydromorphone). Hydration and straining the urine for stones are the mainstays of treatment. Larger stones or suspected infections require urologic consultation.

Cholelithiasis

Presentation: Cholelithiasis (gallstones) typically presents as colicky right upper quadrant pain exacerbated by fatty meals. The pneumonic of the five F's often applies: the patient is "female, fat, forty, fair (white), and fertile." Pain may radiate to the right flank, back, or shoulders.

Examination: Examination usually reveals tenderness in the right upper quadrant. With deeper palpation, as the patient inhales, there may be an abrupt halt in inspiration due to discomfort (Murphy sign). Visceral pain is usual, but peritoneal signs may develop if there is significant inflammation or infection, as in cholecystitis and cholangitis.

Labs may include abnormal liver enzymes (AST, ALT, alkaline phosphatase, bilirubin), but this is highly variable. CBC and UA are normal in uncomplicated cases. Plain films typically are normal, particularly when infection is absent. A right upper quadrant ultrasound or CT scan may reveal stones in the gallbladder or common bile duct. MRI of the gallbladder and ducts (MRCP) may also be helpful. A HIDA scan may be helpful if the above results are equivocal.

Treatment: Medical treatment consists of analgesics, and antibiotics (such as cefotetan, ceftizoxime, and metronidazole) if infection is suspected. However, surgery is the definitive treatment in cholelithiasis. Stones sometimes may be removed through endoscopy.

Peptic Disease

Presentation: Peptic disease usually presents as epigastric or substernal discomfort, which may be made worse (or better) with meals. Reflux of acid after meals or while supine suggests gastroesophageal reflux disease. Ulcers or gastritis/esophagitis and cancer may cause hematemesis (vomiting blood) or melena (black, tarry stools). Other potentially worrisome historical features include early meal satiety, unexplained anemia, weight loss, and dysphagia.

Examination: The exam may be normal, or there may be epigastric tenderness to palpation. Laboratory data such as CBC and UA typically is normal. If there is bleeding, a microcytic anemia, low-serum iron, and positive stool guaiac are common. *Heliobacter pylori* antibodies or stool antigens may be positive. An upper GI series may reveal reflux or ulcers.

Treatment: Treatment usually consists of an H2 blocker or a proton pump inhibitor. Antibiotics are often indicated if the patient has *H. pylori* infection to eradicate the presence of this bacterium. If malignancy is suspected, upper endoscopy is indicated.

Acute Diverticulitis

Presentation: Diverticulitis is more common in patients over the age of 40. Signs and symptoms of infection very similar to appendicitis may be present. Typically, there is a predominance of left-sided symptoms as diverticular disease usually involves the descending colon and sigmoid colon. Fever, abdominal pain, and an elevated WBC may be present, but their frequency varies significantly. Initial visceral pain may progress to overt peritonitis.

Examination: CBC may reveal a normal or elevated WBC. Other labs are not necessary. As with appendicitis, perforation may be evident on plain films, showing subdiaphragmatic free air. CT scanning is helpful in identifying the location and extent of disease.

Treatment: Treatment of diverticulitis includes antibiotics (in combinations such as ciprofloxacin with metronidazole or trimethoprim-sulfamethoxazole with metronidazole), bowel rest, and analgesics. Intravenous antibiotics are indicated if there is evidence of serious infection. Surgery or CT-guided drainage of abscess may be necessary if perforation occurs.

REFERENCES

American College of Emergency Physicians. Clinical policy: Critical issues for the initial evaluation and management of patients presenting with a chief complaint of nontraumatic acute abdominal pain. Ann Emerg Med 2000;36:4.

Carrico CW, Fenton LZ, Taylor GA, et al. Impact of sonography on the diagnosis and treatment of acute lower abdominal pain in children and young adults. Am J Roentgenol 1999;172:513–516.

Esses D, Birnbaum A, Bijur P, et al. Ability of CT to alter decision making in elderly patients with acute abdominal pain. Am J Emerg Med 2004;22(4); 270–272.

Ferozco LB, Raptopoulos V, Silen W. Acute diverticulitis. N Engl J Med 1998;38:1521–1526.

Graff LG, Robinson R. Abdominal pain and emergency department evaluation. Emerg Med Clin North Am 2001;19(1):123–136.

Kamin RA, Nowicki TA, Courtney DS, Powers RD. Pearls and pitfalls in the emergency department evaluation of abdominal pain. Emerg Med Clin North Am 2003;21(1):61–72.

Leung AK, Sigalet DL. Acute abdominal pain in children. Am Fam Physician 2003;7:2321–2326.

Trowbridge RL, Rutkowski NK, Shojania KG. Does this patient have acute cholecystitis? JAMA 2003; 289:80–86.

Wagner JM, McKinney P, Carpenter JL. Does this patient have appendicitis? JAMA 1996; 276:1589–1594.

Weyant MJ, Barie PS, Eachempati SR. Clinical role of noncontrast helical computed tomography in diagnosis of acute appendicitis. Am J Surg 2002; 183(1):97–99.

"I'm Worried about Grandpa"

Examinee Prompt

You are seeing this elderly male patient in your primary care office for an evaluation of weight loss. Please complete the following tasks:

- ❑ Obtain a focused history relevant to the chief complaint.
- ❑ Conduct an appropriate physical examination.
- ❑ During the examination, please state what you are examining.

You have 15 minutes to complete your visit with the patient. When you have all of the information that you need you may leave the examination room. You do not need to explain your findings to the patient. Following your visit with the patient, you will be asked to write a complete progress note using the "SOAP" (Subjective, Objective, Assessment, and Plan) format. Please include an assessment as well as a five-item differential diagnosis and as a diagnostic/treatment plan. You will have 10 additional minutes to complete the progress note.

If there are any portions of the examination that you would normally perform, please state them to the patient. If there is any portion of the examination that the model patient does not want examined, he or she may state the findings of that portion of the examination.

Vital Signs

Temperature .... 97.5°F
Blood pressure 103/50
Heart rate 70
Respiratory rate 12
Height .... 5′10″
Weight .... 160 pounds
Body mass index 23

Patient Prompt

Background: You are playing the role of a 71-year-old man who was sent to the doctor by family members. The family is concerned about your recent progressive weight loss.

Chief Complaint: "I'm losing weight and don't know why."

History of the Present Illness: 71-year-old man who first noticed unintentional weight loss about 8 to 9 months ago when clothing began to feel looser. More recently your family had a party and they all voiced their concern. Though you almost never visit the doctor, the entire family insisted that you come in for evaluation. "They all think I'm dying of cancer." You are much less concerned.

You do not routinely weigh yourself, but you are fairly sure that your normal weight is between 180 and 185 pounds. Just prior to your visit, your weight was 160 pounds.

Past Medical History: None known (you haven't been to a doctor in at least 35 to 40 years).

Past Surgical History:
- Appendectomy at age 14
- Surgery for a gunshot wound to the leg in the Korean War

Allergies: No known drug allergies

Medications: None

Social History:
- Retired car mechanic
- Lives with wife
- Four adult children and three grandchildren
- Expecting your first great-grandchild
- Drinks three to four mixed drinks per day
- Quit smoking 20 years ago (50 pack-year smoking history)

Review of Systems:
- No fevers or chills
- No nausea or vomiting
- Your appetite has been poor for the last year or so
- You deny poor dentition or difficulty swallowing
- No early satiety
- No abdominal pain or change in bowel habit
- No melena or bright red blood per rectum
- You have an occasional cough, which is nonproductive
- No hemoptysis
- No shortness of breath, chest pain, palpitations, or anginal symptoms
- No paroxysmal nocturnal dyspnea or orthopnea
- No depressive symptoms

- No heat or cold intolerance
- No skin, hair, or nail changes
- Review of systems is otherwise negative

Additional Information:

- During the examination, the examiner will state what he or she is examining.
- The examiner should not perform a rectal exam on the standardized patient.
- All portions of this physical examination are intended to be normal.

Geriatric Weight Loss Scoresheet

Subjective

- ❑ Asks chief complaint
- ❑ Weight loss quantified (or asks previous weight and compares to current weight)
- ❑ Asks about diet
- ❑ Constitutional symptoms (fevers, chills, anorexia)
- ❑ Gastrointestinal symptoms (any three of the following: dentition issues, swallowing difficulties, nausea, vomiting, change in bowel habits, abdominal pain, bloating, gastrointestinal bleeding)
- ❑ Pulmonary symptoms (any two of the following: cough, hemoptysis, shortness of breath, dyspnea on exertion, or other pulmonary symptoms)
- ❑ Cardiac symptoms (any two of the following: chest pain, shortness of breath, palpitations, jaw/arm pain, paroxysmal nocturnal dyspnea, orthopnea)
- ❑ Depressive symptoms
- ❑ Past medical history
- ❑ Smoking history in pack years
- ❑ Alcohol use
- ❑ Previous medical evaluations

Objective

- ❑ General assessment
- ❑ Documents any temporal or thenar wasting
- ❑ Examines and comments on dentition
- ❑ Adenopathy
- ❑ Skin lesions
- ❑ Cardiac examination
- ❑ Pulmonary examination
- ❑ Abdominal examination

Assessment/Differential Diagnosis

- ❑ Elderly male with unintentional weight loss
- ❑ Differential diagnosis should include five of the following: lung cancer, colon cancer, prostate cancer, gastrointestinal etiologies, depression, alcohol abuse, hyperthyroidism

Plan

- ❑ Rectal exam
- ❑ Credit for up to five of the following: complete blood count (CBC), thyroid-stimulating hormone (TSH), urinalysis, electrolytes, blood urea nitrogen (BUN) and creatinine, liver function tests, chest x-ray or computed tomography (CT) scan of chest, CT scan of abdomen, fecal occult blood testing, prostate-specific antigen (PSA), albumin or prealbumin, nutritionist evaluation, trial of hypercaloric feeding supplements

Total Score: ____ / 31

Passing score for this station is 21 correct items.

Communication and Interpersonal Skills (CIS) Scoresheet

Please rate each of the following items on a scale from 1–10.
These items may be completed by either the standardized patient or another student.

Scoresheet 1

	Poor		Fair		Good		Very Good		Excellent	
Professional appearance	1	2	3	4	5	6	7	8	9	10
Introduces self and shakes hands	1	2	3	4	5	6	7	8	9	10
Nonverbal communication (eye contact, facial expressiveness, body language)	1	2	3	4	5	6	7	8	9	10
Communicates effectively (open-ended questions, avoids jargon)	1	2	3	4	5	6	7	8	9	10
Establishes rapport with patient (empathy, appears nonjudgmental)	1	2	3	4	5	6	7	8	9	10
Allows patient to speak without being interrupted	1	2	3	4	5	6	7	8	9	10
Listens and seems to understand patient's concerns	1	2	3	4	5	6	7	8	9	10
Overall professionalism	1	2	3	4	5	6	7	8	9	10

Total Score:

Passing score for CIS section is 56 points.

Spoken English Proficiency (SEP) Scoresheet

Please rate each of the following items on a scale from 1–10.
These items may be completed by either the standardized patient or another student.

Scoresheet 2

	Poor		Fair		Good		Very Good		Excellent	
Examiner is articulate and easily understood	1	2	3	4	5	6	7	8	9	10
Pronunciation (words pronounced correctly; accent does not hinder communication)	1	2	3	4	5	6	7	8	9	10
Word choice is appropriate	1	2	3	4	5	6	7	8	9	10
Ability to communicate without excessive listener effort required to understand questions or responses	1	2	3	4	5	6	7	8	9	10
Patient's ability to understand the examiner	1	2	3	4	5	6	7	8	9	10
Examiner's ability to understand the patient	1	2	3	4	5	6	7	8	9	10

Total Score:

Passing score for SEP section is 42 points.

Evaluation and Management of Geriatric Weight Loss

Overview

An elderly patient with involuntary or unintentional weight loss can be anxiety provoking for the patient, the patient's family, and the physician. For the family, a common concern is the possibility of cancer as the cause of the weight loss. For the physician, a broad differential diagnosis, the potential difficulty in obtaining an accurate history, the possibility of missing elderly neglect, and the concern that a cancer may be overlooked all may cause anxiety.

Involuntary weight loss is associated with a significant increase in morbidity and mortality in the elderly population. The differential diagnosis of weight loss is cumbersome and virtually endless. Rather than focus on a long list of potential causes, this chapter provides a systematic approach to the topic of geriatric weight loss, which intends to make accurate diagnosis and effective management easier to achieve.

Initial Evaluation and Screening

The initial evaluation, as with most problems, begins with a detailed history. Time limitations and impaired cognitive function can make this more difficult, but starting with the most common etiologies first (with a focused history and physical) may streamline the workup. The "shotgun" approach, the indiscriminate ordering of numerous diagnostic studies, should be reserved for unique situations in which the clinical suspicion for underlying malignancy is high or the ability to obtain a sufficient history is inadequate.

A patient's past medical history is particularly important in the diagnostic evaluation. Quantification of weight loss is essential by serial documentation of the patient's weight in the medical record. In some cases, the patient may provide an accurate history of past weight, which can be compared with the present.

The history and physical examination should be thorough but with a focus on several of the most common causes of weight loss:

- Malignancy. The most common malignancies in the elderly population are lung, breast, prostate, and colorectal cancers. The patient's smoking history, date and findings of the most recent mammogram, date and findings of the last colonoscopy, and any recent chest x-rays should be reviewed. Additionally the patient should be asked about any respiratory complaint. A thorough examination should be performed, including a breast exam, pelvic exam, rectal exam, and prostate exam.
- Psychiatric causes. Depression may present atypically, sometimes with weight loss as the presenting symptom.
- Gastrointestinal problems. Oral and dental problems (poor dentition, dentures that do not fit correctly), swallowing problems, inability to feed oneself, constipation, and biliary stones may contribute to weight loss. A review of systems should focus on caloric intake, anorexia, quantification of weight loss, nausea, abdominal pain, bloating, voiding habits, rectal bleeding, and melena.
- Medications. Side effects, as well as issues of polypharmacy may result in weight loss. Having the patient bring all of his or her medications to the doctor's visit is recommended. Any medication changes coinciding with the onset of weight loss are also helpful to note. In addition to prescription medications, all over-the-counter medications and any supplements should also be considered.

Diagnostic Tests

If the history and physical examination do not suggest a particular diagnosis for the cause of the weight loss, initial screening labs usually are indicated. The following list provides commonly ordered studies in the evaluation of weight loss:

1. CBC (looking for anemia or decreased total lymphocyte count)
2. TSH
3. Urinalysis (proteinuria may result in loss of nutrients and antibodies)
4. Serum chemistry profile
    - Electrolytes
    - BUN and creatinine
    - Blood glucose
    - Calcium
    - Liver function tests (aspartate transaminase [AST], alanine transaminase [ALT], alkaline phosphatase, lactate dehydrogenase, bilirubin)
    - Amylase and lipase
5. PSA
6. Stool occult blood testing
7. Purified protein derivative (PPD) if risk factors are present
8. Human immunodeficiency virus (HIV) if risk factors are present

9. Chest x-ray (may reveal a mass, cardiomegaly/congestive heart failure, infiltrate or adenopathy)
10. Mammogram

If lung cancer is suspected on the basis of symptomatology or a smoking history, a CT scan of the chest and/or bronchoscopy should be considered.

If a gastrointestinal problem is suspected, an upper and/or lower endoscopy should be considered based on the suspected diagnosis. A CT scan of the abdomen may be indicated when certain abdominal processes are suspected.

If diarrhea is an associated symptom, consider screening for celiac sprue with anti-gliadin and anti-endomysial antibodies.

If a hematologic malignancy is suspected, a peripheral smear of the blood, a serum protein electrophoresis (SPEP), and possibly a bone marrow biopsy may be helpful.

Nutritional Assessment

In some cases it is possible to identify an underlying etiology for a patient's weight loss despite a thorough diagnostic evaluation. A comprehensive nutritional assessment, often performed by a trained nutritionist, may provide valuable information. It is clear that adequate nutrition is essential to maintenance of health, as well as recovery from acute and chronic illness. Though calorie counts and the various elements of a nutrition assessment are beyond the scope of this chapter, there are several basic principles that should be discussed:

- Cachexia vs. starvation. Cachexia is weight loss caused by an underlying disease, due to abnormally high levels of tumor necrosis factor (cachectin) or interleukin-1β, interleukin-6, and adipsia. It is valuable, therefore, to distinguish cachexia from starvation, which is simply restricted caloric intake. There are numerous systemic diseases that can cause cachexia, and there are equally many factors that can lead to starvation. If a clinician is able to determine which of the two is present, the remainder of the diagnostic evaluation may then be narrowed. The treatment of the weight loss also differs significantly, as cachexia is relatively unresponsive to increased caloric intake. In fact, a poor response to increased caloric intake may suggest cachexia.
- There is certain laboratory data and other information that is pertinent to a nutritional assessment:

1. Body Mass Index (BMI) or free fat mass.
2. Albumin or prealbumin. (Serum albumin is decreased with malnutrition but may be increased with certain disease states as an acute phase reactant.)
3. Total lymphocyte count. The total white blood cell count multiplied by the percentage of lymphocytes equals the total lymphocyte count. Total lymphocyte count may be decreased in malnutrition, but may be elevated in acute illness.
4. Cholesterol levels may be low, especially with cachexia.
5. Calorie counts are valuable in determining the degree of intake.
6. Weight trend (10 pounds in 6 months is considered significant).
7. Adequacy of intake (<50% eaten of regular meals is significant).

Treatment

Obviously, the treatment of weight loss is focused on determining an underlying etiology and treating or curing that problem. However, in many elderly patients, a cause for the weight loss cannot be determined despite an extensive evaluation. In these cases, there are several ways to treat the weight loss.

Consider Removing All Dietary Restrictions

If a patient is on a special diet for medical reasons, strongly consider removing these restrictions. Malnutrition alone can lead to a significant increased morbidity and mortality. Therefore the risks of removing the restrictions may be outweighed by the constitutional benefits.

Hypercaloric Feeding

Following a complete evaluation by a physician and an assessment by a nutritionist, a decision may be made to provide the patient with caloric supplementation. There are numerous brands of supplements that provide a relatively dense source of calories. Selection usually is made on the basis of patient preference, though certain underlying medical conditions may affect the choice.

Medications

- Cyproheptadine is a sedating antihistamine. Because of the significant side-effect profile of this medication, its use is quite limited.
- Steroids. Glucocorticoids can decrease the hormonal mediators of cachexia but also have

significant potential side effects. Anabolic steroids may be of benefit, depending upon the underlying disease.

- Testosterone. Replacement of low testosterone has shown to be of benefit by increasing muscle mass and strength.
- Megestrol is a progestin that stimulates appetite and inhibits various cytokines. Although it is effective, it should be used with caution in patients with a high risk of deep venous thrombosis.
- Dronabinol is a synthetic form of tetrahydrocannabinol (THC) that can stimulate appetite and reduce nausea. It can also have several other favorable effects on a patient, such as better mood, decrease in pain, and improved taste and smell. This is a controlled substance that is quite expensive.
- Mirtazapine is an antidepressant that can cause weight gain.

REFERENCES

Aisner J, Parnes H, Tait N, et al. Appetite stimulation and weight gain with megestrol acetate. Semin Oncol 1990;17(6 suppl 9):2–7.

Fawcett J, Barkin RL. Review of the results from clinical studies on the efficacy, safety and tolerability of mirtazapine for the treatment of patients with major depression. J Affect Disord 1998;51(3):267–285.

Gazewood JD, Mehr DR. Diagnosis and management of weight loss in the elderly. J Fam Pract 1998;47:19–25.

Guigoz Y, Vellas B, Garry PJ. Assessing the nutritional status of the elderly: The Mini Nutritional Assessment as part of the geriatric evaluation. Nutr Rev 1996;54:S59–S65.

Hernández JL, Riancho JA, Matorras P, González-Macías J. Clinical evaluation for cancer in patients with involuntary weight loss without specific symptoms. Am J Med 2003;114(8):631–637.

Holister LE. Hunger and appetite after single doses of marijuana, alcohol, and dextroamphetamine. Clin Pharmacol Ther 1971;12(1):44–49.

Huffman GB. Evaluating and treating unintentional weight loss in the elderly. Am Fam Physician 2002;65:640–650.

Morley JE. Anorexia of aging: Physiologic and pathologic. Am J Clin Nutr 1997;66:760–773.

Morley JE. Anorexia in older persons: Epidemiology and optimal treatment. Drugs Aging 1996;8(2):134–155.

Morley JE. Orexigenic and anabolic agents. Clin Geriatr Med 2002;18(4):853–866.

Reife CM. Involuntary weight loss. Med Clin North Am 1995;79:299–313.

Thompson MP, Morris LK. Unexplained weight loss in the ambulatory elderly. J Am Geriatr Soc 1991;39:497–500.

Verdery RB. Clinical evaluation of failure to thrive in older people. Clin Geriatr Med 1997;13:769–778.

Wise GR, Craig D. Evaluation of involuntary weight loss. Where do you start? Postgrad Med 1994;95:143–146.

"My Back Is Killing Me"

Examinee Prompt

You are seeing this 43-year-old patient in your office for a chief complaint of "low back pain." Please complete the following tasks:

- ❑ Obtain a focused history relevant to this patient's complaint.
- ❑ Perform an appropriate physical examination.
- ❑ Explain your findings and plan to the patient.

You have 15 minutes to complete your visit with the patient. Following your visit with the patient, you will have 10 minutes to complete a progress note in the standard "SOAP" (Subjective, Objective, Assessment and Plan) format.

Vital Signs

Temperature .... 98.8°F

Blood pressure .... 135/75 mm Hg

Pulse 82

Respiratory rate 12

Patient Prompt

Background: 43-year-old patient with 2-day history of low back pain. You have had a few episodes of back pain in the past, but nothing very significant. This episode seems to be worse than the others. You have heard of "slipped disks" and want to be sure that this has not happened to you.

Chief Complaint: Low back pain

History of the Present Illness: 43-year-old patient with 2-day history of low back pain. Pain began 2 days ago after playing flag football with the family at Thanksgiving. This consisted of fairly strenuous activity, but there was no trauma. The pain is deep and aching and is most significant in the right lower back. The pain does not radiate down the legs. There are no obvious exacerbating or alleviating factors. There is no extremity weakness or numbness and no bowel or bladder incontinence. Ibuprofen 400 mg every 8 hours has not provided significant relief.

Past Medical History: Gout

Past Surgical History: Left knee arthroscopy for a torn meniscus

Gynecologic History:
- Not applicable if male.
- If female, no pregnancies.
- LMP 2 weeks ago.

Medications: Allopurinol 100 mg daily

Allergies: Cephalosporins, which cause facial swelling

Family History: Father has lung cancer. Mother has had "minor strokes."

Social History:
- Married, 2 children
- Advertising executive
- Quit smoking 10 years ago, 10 pack-year smoking history
- Drink alcohol socially only

Review of Systems:
- No fever, no weight loss
- No headache, no visual changes
- No chest pain, shortness of breath, cough, or hemoptysis
- No abdominal pain, diarrhea, constipation, melena, or bright red blood per rectum
- No groin pain
- No dysuria, hematuria, or urgency

Additional Information: During the examination, please attempt to "act out" the following clinical signs:

- Range of motion is partially limited during flexion due to discomfort.
- Tenderness to palpation in the lumbar paraspinal musculature, more on the right side than the left side.
- No bony tenderness to palpation.
- Gait is normal.
- Straight leg raise test is negative.
- Sensation is intact.
- Deep tendon reflexes are normal (you may state this when the examiner performs the test).
- Peripheral muscle strength is normal throughout.

Scoring Sheet

Subjective

- ❑ Onset of pain
- ❑ Location of pain
- ❑ Radiation of pain
- ❑ Exacerbating and alleviating factors
- ❑ Previous history of back problems or back trauma
- ❑ Fever
- ❑ Weight loss
- ❑ Past medical history

Objective

- ❑ Visual inspection
- ❑ Palpation of bony structures and musculature
- ❑ Range of motion
- ❑ Assessment of gait
- ❑ Straight leg raise
- ❑ Assessment of deep tendon reflexes
- ❑ Assessment of peripheral sensation
- ❑ Assessment of muscle strength

Assessment

- ❑ Axial low back pain (any of the following are acceptable: muscular low back pain, ligamentous injury, degenerative changes, or facet joint dysfunction). Disk herniation is not acceptable.

Plan

- ❑ Limited rest or activity modification
- ❑ Nonsteroidal anti-inflammatory medication
- ❑ Indicates a follow-up appointment or the importance of returning for reevaluation if symptoms do not improve

The following evaluations are not appropriate, and one point should be deducted for each:

- ❑ Magnetic resonance imaging (MRI) for the initial evaluation
- ❑ Bone scan
- ❑ Computed tomography (CT) scan

Total Score: ____ / 20

Passing score for this station is 14 correct items.

Communication and Interpersonal Skills (CIS) Scoresheet

Please rate each of the following items on a scale from 1–10.
These items may be completed by either the standardized patient or another student.

Scoresheet 1

	Poor		Fair		Good		Very Good		Excellent	
Professional appearance	1	2	3	4	5	6	7	8	9	10
Introduces self and shakes hands	1	2	3	4	5	6	7	8	9	10
Nonverbal communication (eye contact, facial expressiveness, body language)	1	2	3	4	5	6	7	8	9	10
Communicates effectively (open-ended questions, avoids jargon)	1	2	3	4	5	6	7	8	9	10
Establishes rapport with patient (empathy, appears nonjudgmental)	1	2	3	4	5	6	7	8	9	10
Allows patient to speak without being interrupted	1	2	3	4	5	6	7	8	9	10
Listens and seems to understand patient's concerns	1	2	3	4	5	6	7	8	9	10
Overall professionalism	1	2	3	4	5	6	7	8	9	10

Total Score:

Passing score for CIS section is 56 points.

Spoken English Proficiency (SEP) Scoresheet

Please rate each of the following items on a scale from 1–10.
These items may be completed by either the standardized patient or another student.

Scoresheet 2

	Poor		Fair		Good		Very Good		Excellent	
Examiner is articulate and easily understood	1	2	3	4	5	6	7	8	9	10
Pronunciation (words pronounced correctly; accent does not hinder communication)	1	2	3	4	5	6	7	8	9	10
Word choice is appropriate	1	2	3	4	5	6	7	8	9	10
Ability to communicate without excessive listener effort required to understand questions or responses	1	2	3	4	5	6	7	8	9	10
Patient's ability to understand the examiner	1	2	3	4	5	6	7	8	9	10
Examiner's ability to understand the patient	1	2	3	4	5	6	7	8	9	10

Total Score:

Passing score for SEP section is 42 points.

The Approach to the Patient with Acute Low Back Pain

Anatomy

There are five lumbar vertebrae, and each is composed of a body, two pedicles, two laminae, four articular facets, and a spinous process. Between each pair of vertebrae are the foramina. Through these openings pass the spinal nerve root, the radicular blood vessels, and sinuvertebral nerves. The spinal canal is formed by the laminae and ligamentum flavum posteriorly, the vertebral bodies and intervertebral disks anteriorly, and the pedicles anterolaterally.

The facet joints are true synovial joints, and are subject to degenerative and inflammatory change. Facet arthropathy can contribute to radicular pain. Chronic degenerative and inflammatory change can result in joint enlargement and thickening of the ligamentum flavum, which can contribute to canal stenosis.

The intervertebral disk provides support for the column of vertebral bones while maintaining elasticity to permit the required mobility of the spine. Each intervertebral disk is composed of a ring of the annulus fibrosus, which is a ring of elastic collagen surrounding the gelatinous nucleus pulposus. As the disk ages or becomes chronically injured, the amount of fibrous tissue increases and gradually replaces the elastic collagen fibers. The disk becomes less elastic, and over time becomes fissured. Ultimately, the disk deteriorates into a desiccated, fragmented annulus fibrosus surrounding a fibrotic nucleus pulposus. Controversy exists over the exact mechanism of pain, but the degenerating disk is a common source of axial somatic pain.

Numerous ligaments are responsible for vertebral stability and, along with the paraspinous muscles, help to control and limit spinal column motion. The posterior ligament forms the anterior wall of the spinal canal, and narrows gradually as it extends inferiorly. This narrowing makes it susceptible to injury and disk herniation, particularly at the lower lumbar levels. The ligamentum flavum spans the space between the laminae, and with age it can thicken and contribute to lumbar stenosis.

The paraspinous muscles are responsible for maintaining erect posture and participate in many of the motions of the spinal column. These muscles are the principal source of pain in many cases of acute low back pain.

Pathophysiology

Acute low back pain can be divided into three main categories for the purposes of evaluation and treatment: (1) axial, (2) radicular, and (3) referred.

Axial pain is caused by noxious stimuli affecting nerve endings in the annular outer portion of the disks, vertebral end plates, and facet joints. Causes of axial pain include muscular strains, ligamentous injuries, facet joint dysfunction, and degenerative changes in the spine. Patients with axial pain describe their back pain as deep, aching, and diffuse. Derangements of the intervertebral disk and increased tension in the paraspinous muscles are the most common causes of axial somatic pain. Though axial pain usually does not radiate, pain from the facet joint may cause back pain and referred leg pain.

Radicular back pain is caused by compression of a nerve root, causing lancinating or shooting pain with extension in a distinct band down the lower extremity. The most frequent cause of radicular pain is disk herniation, though it is also caused by foraminal or lateral recess stenosis. Stenosis of the foramen or lateral recess can be caused by facet arthropathy and osteophyte formation, ligamentous hypertrophy, and spondylolisthesis. The term *sciatica* refers to radiating pain in either lower extremity distal to the knee. Sciatica is associated most commonly with L5 and S1 radiculopathies, which together comprise more than 90% of all lumbosacral radiculopathies.

Referred pain can be caused by many processes affecting the organs of the abdomen and retroperitoneum. These processes include abdominal aortic aneurysm, renal colic, organomegaly, or tumors of abdominal organs.

History

The principal purpose of obtaining the history in low back pain is to identify the small percentage of patients with serious conditions who require immediate further evaluation and intervention. These serious conditions include malignancy, infection, neurologic disorders, and rheumatologic diseases.

The history should include the following components:

- Patient age
- Onset of pain (e.g., certain activities, time of day)
- History of trauma
- Type and character of pain (e.g., sharp, dull, achy)
- Location of pain (e.g., unilateral, bilateral, midline)
- Radiation of pain (how far down the leg does the pain radiate?)
- Exacerbating and alleviating factors (coughing and sneezing may exacerbate pain due to

disk herniation). Radicular pain may be reduced in the supine position and is worsened by standing or sitting.

- Symptoms of claudication
- Neurologic symptoms such as numbness, weakness, bowel and bladder dysfunction
- Visceral pain
- Past medical history, including previous back injuries or surgeries
- Previous therapy for back pain and its efficacy
- Psychosocial stressors
- Fever
- Weight loss

Examination

Before actually examining the patient, the clinician should check for fever, which may suggest the presence of an underlying infection such as osteomyelitis, diskitis, or an epidural abscess.

The physical examination should begin with a visual inspection of the back for any deformity. A prominent spinous process may indicate the presence of spondylolisthesis, which is the forward slippage of a vertebra on the one below it. The patient who is bending forward and has difficulty straightening up may have a large central disk derangement. Any scoliosis should be noted. The level of the two iliac crests should be noted by palpating them simultaneously as any unevenness may indicate a leg length discrepancy.

In addition to evaluating the physical structures of the back, specific attention should be given to the skin. Certain disorders such as psoriasis, neurofibromatosis, and herpes zoster may be associated with low back pain.

Tenderness should be elicited by palpation both along the musculature and the bony structure of the low back. A muscle strain may produce tenderness over the involved musculature. In the patient with radiation of low back pain, tenderness may be elicited over the sciatic notch. Tenderness over the sacroiliac joints can be a sign of spondylitis.

Range of motion should be evaluated by having the patient flex, extend, tilt laterally, and rotate the torso at the hips. Pain with flexion is common in disk derangements, and deviation to one side with forward flexion may indicate a posterolateral disk bulge. Extension while standing can alleviate the pain of a disk derangement, though it may actually be irritating in the early course of disk derangements. Localized pain in the lumbar or paralumbar region associated with extension may indicate a facet syndrome.

A straight leg raise test should be performed in all patients complaining of low back pain (Figure 1). With the patient in the supine position, the leg is raised straight up. The test is considered positive if radiating pain occurs when the leg is elevated between 30 and 70 degrees of elevation. Radiating pain is the result of stretching a pinched nerve root, usually as a result of disk herniation. The contralateral straight leg raise test is positive when a straight leg raise test in the asymptomatic leg causes radiating pain in the symptomatic leg.

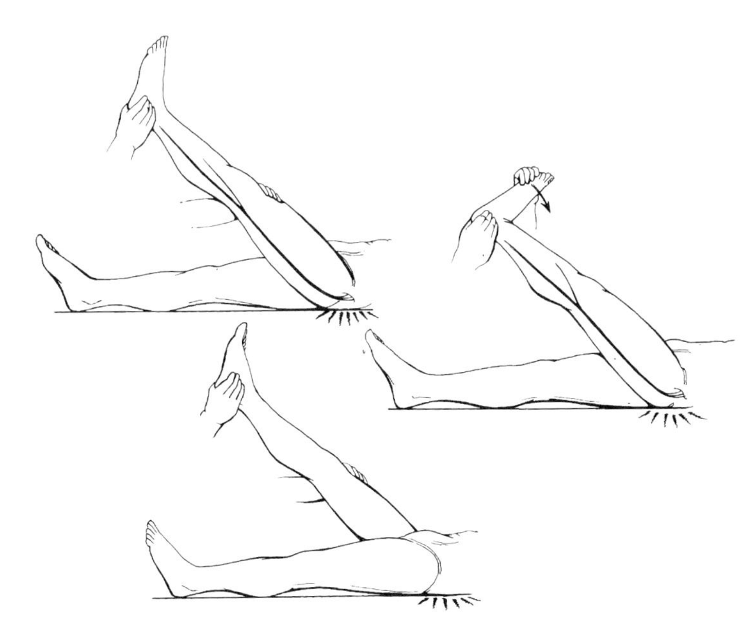

Figure 1. Straight leg test. (From DeLee J, Drez D, Miller MD. DeLee and Drez's Orthopaedic Sports Medicine, 2nd ed. Philadelphia, Elsevier, 2003, fig. 27 A(7), with permission.)

A thorough neurologic examination should be performed in all patients with low back pain and should consist of the following components:

- Gait assessment. The patient should be assessed for an antalgic gait favoring one leg. Any footdrop should be considered significant.
- Motor testing. Heel walking, toe walking, hopping on either foot, or toe tapping may reveal evidence of weakness and suggest a radiculopathy. The distribution of weakness within a particular myotome should be noted.
- Sensory testing. The patient should be evaluated for evidence of sensory loss within a given dermatome.
- Reflexes. Cremasteric, thigh adductor, patellar, and Achilles reflexes should be evaluated.

If the patient complains of pain radiating to the hip or buttock, the hip should be thoroughly examined. Degenerative joint disease and occult hip fractures can cause pain in the ipsilateral buttock and low back.

An abdominal examination is an important part of the evaluation in all patients with low back pain. The abdominal examination may reveal causes of referred pain such as abdominal aortic aneurysm, renal colic, organomegaly, or tumors of abdominal organs.

Evaluation and Treatment

The goal of the evaluation of the patient with low back pain should be to exclude the rare conditions that require early aggressive intervention while using a symptom-directed approach to diagnosis and treatment. The two major conditions to be ruled out are cauda equina syndrome and progressive muscle weakness. If either of these conditions is suspected on clinical grounds, an MRI should be performed immediately. If the results of the MRI confirm the diagnosis, immediate surgical decompression of the offending lesion should be performed.

Plain-film radiography is rarely useful in the initial evaluation of patients with acute-onset low back pain. Several large studies have demonstrated

Table 1

Differential Diagnosis of Low Back Pain

Differential Diagnosis of Low Back Pain
Back strain (muscular, ligamentous)
Acute disk herniation
Osteoarthritis or spinal stenosis
Ankylosing spondylitis
Malignancy
Primary tumor
Metastatic tumor
Carcinomatous meningitis
Infection
Osteomyelitis
Epidural abscess
Tuberculosis
HIV infection
Herpes zoster
Lyme disease
Inflammatory disorders
Sarcoidosis
Vasculitis
Traumatic disorders
Disk herniation
Vertebral fracture
Endocrine and metabolic disorders
Diabetic retinopathy
Vertebral fracture (due to osteoporosis, malignancy, etc.)
Acromegaly
Paget disease
Congenital and developmental disorders
Spondylolisthesis
Synovial cyst
Arteriovenous malformation

the low yield of lumbar spine radiographs in the acute setting. However, radiographs should be considered in patients who meet any of the following criteria:

- History of significant trauma
- Neurologic deficits
- Fever
- Unexplained weight loss
- Systemic symptoms that suggest infection or malignancy
- History of cancer, corticosteroid use, immunodeficient state, or drug or alcohol abuse
- Ankylosing spondylitis suspected

In patients with worsening neurologic deficits or a suspected systemic cause of back pain such as infection or malignancy, MRI or CT scan should be considered.

In most cases of low back pain of suspected axial or radicular etiology, activity modification and nonsteroidal anti-inflammatory medications are the hallmark of therapy. For severe pain, short-term use of a narcotic may be considered. If symptoms fail to resolve within the first few weeks, physical therapy focusing on range of motion and muscular strengthening exercises may provide benefit. If symptoms persist beyond 4 to 6 weeks, radiographs are indicated to rule out spondylolysis, spondylolisthesis, occult compression fracture, occult infection, or malignancy.

For patients with radicular symptoms who fail to respond to conservative therapy, an MRI may be considered. These patients may benefit from an epidural steroid injection, which serves both diagnostic and therapeutic purposes. In some of these patients, surgical evaluation for a diskectomy may be necessary. In the patient with predominantly radicular symptoms and a normal MRI, a workup for peripheral neuropathy should be considered.

For patients with persistent axial complaints despite adequate medical and physical therapy, the clinician should reconsider the diagnosis and treatment plan. The patient may require a workup for gastrointestinal, genitourinary, hematologic, or biochemical abnormalities. In these patients, MRI may be useful to rule out occult tumor or infection. However, it must be considered that many asymptomatic individuals have disk derangements, so a disk abnormality should not necessarily be considered the source of pain in the patient with axial complaints.

REFERENCES

Devereaux MW. Low back pain. Primary Care Clin Office Pract 2004;31:33–51.

Dulaney E. Radiculopathy and cauda equina syndrome. In: Evans RW, ed. Saunders Manual of Neurologic Practice. Philadelphia, Elsevier, 2003, pp 757–763.

Jensen MC, Brant-Zawadzki MN, Obuchowski N, et al. Magnetic resonance imaging of the lumbar spine in people without back pain. N Engl J Med 1994;331:69–73.

Levin KH, Covington EC, Devereaux MW, et al. Neck and low back pain. Continuum 2001;7:1–205.

Patel AT, Ogle AA. Diagnosis and management of acute low back pain. Am Fam Physician 2000;61:1779–1786.

Porter RW, Ralston SH. Pharmacological management of back pain syndromes. Drugs 1994;48:189–198.

Scavone JG, Latshaw RF, Rohrer GV. Use of lumbar spine films. Statistical evaluation at a university teaching hospital. JAMA 1981;246:1105–1108.

Scavone JG, Latshaw RF, Weidner WA. Anteroposterior and lateral radiographs: An adequate lumbar spine examination. Am J Roentgenol 1981;136:715–717.

"I'm Tired All the Time"

Examinee Prompt

While working in an outpatient clinic, you are asked to see this 28-year-old patient for a complaint of fatigue. Please complete the following tasks:

- Obtain a focused history relevant to this patient's complaint.
- Perform an appropriate physical examination.
- Discuss your diagnosis and plan with the patient.

You will have 15 minutes to complete your visit with the patient. When you have completed the interaction, you may leave the examination room. You will have 10 additional minutes to complete a progress note using the standard "SOAP" (Subjective, Objective, Assessment and Plan) format.

Vital Signs

Temperature .... 98.2°F

Blood pressure .... 118/68 mm Hg

Pulse 70

Respiratory rate 15

Patient Prompt

Background: You are a 28-year-old patient seeing a doctor today after several of your friends have voiced concern about your behavior. You may offer any of the following information if specifically asked by the examiner.

Chief Complaint: Fatigue

History of the Present Illness: 28-year-old patient with a concern about decreasing energy and poor sleep for the past 2 to 3 months. You have attributed these symptoms to being "stressed out" though you are unable to identify any single dominant stressor. You have both difficulty falling asleep (due to ruminating thoughts or issues that need to be dealt with the following day) as well as difficulty maintaining restful sleep. You are often quite tired in the morning and have called in sick to work because of this. Naps during the day help with your fatigue, but only by about 50%. You often stay up very late watching movies to avoid going to bed.

Your appetite has decreased as well, and you often crave junk food. You are unsure about weight gain, but you "wouldn't be surprised." You have difficulty with concentration, and as a result make many mistakes at work. You have grown less interested in social activities and activities that you once enjoyed (you used to enjoy going to the movies and collecting movie memorabilia). You have significantly less self-esteem as well as nonspecific worries and anxiety.

You deny ever having a panic attack. You do sometimes feel slowed down or "in a fog." You have not had any suicidal ideation. You deny depressed mood but just "don't really feel anything." Your main reason for coming to the doctor is that your friends and family have all voiced concern. You, however, think that everyone is being overly critical. "People say I'm too moody, but I feel like everyone is just giving me a hard time."

Past Medical History: Otherwise healthy

Medications: None

Allergies: No known drug allergies

Social History:

- Single
- You work at a movie rental store
- No significant work stress
- Few close friends (good support network)
- You haven't been interested in social activities or hobbies
- No tobacco
- Minimal alcohol consumption
- You live with one roommate from college
- You had a 1-year romantic relationship that ended 6 months ago

Family History: No family history of mood disorder or psychiatric illness

Review of Systems:

- No shortness of breath, dyspnea on exertion, or exercise intolerance
- No heat or cold intolerance
- No change in hair growth

- No menstrual irregularity (if female)
- No diarrhea, constipation, nausea or vomiting
- No urinary symptoms
- No chest pain or palpitations
- No upper respiratory symptoms
- No hallucinations or other psychotic symptoms

Additional Information: At first during the interview, you are *convinced* that your symptoms are due to a serious medical condition. If the issue of depression is entertained, you are hesitant to accept this because you "don't feel sad." Later, after further explanation, you may accept the diagnosis and treatment options because you "really do want to feel better."

The physical exam is intended to be unremarkable.

Depression Case Scoresheet

Subjective

- ❑ Asks chief complaint
- ❑ Duration of symptoms
- ❑ Level of impairment (work, social, etc.)
- ❑ Sleep (including at least one element such as falling asleep, staying asleep, or difficulty waking up)
- ❑ Appetite
- ❑ Social history (must include use of drug or alcohol use for credit)
- ❑ Concentration
- ❑ Interests
- ❑ Psychomotor symptoms
- ❑ Association of symptoms with menstrual period (if female)
- ❑ Past medical history
- ❑ Medications
- ❑ Allergies
- ❑ Suicidal ideation
- ❑ Weapons available
- ❑ Psychotic features
- ❑ History of manic episodes

Objective

- ❑ Vital signs
- ❑ Examination of the conjunctiva for signs of anemia
- ❑ Examination of the thyroid gland
- ❑ Cardiac exam
- ❑ Pulmonary exam

Diagnosis (credit for up to 2 of the following items)

- ❑ Major depression (Depression also acceptable. Anhedonia is not acceptable.)
- ❑ Hypothyroidism
- ❑ Anemia
- ❑ Secondary depression

Plan (credit for up to 5 of the following items)

- ❑ Offer counseling
- ❑ Discuss possible use of medications
- ❑ Order complete blood count (CBC)
- ❑ Order thyroid-stimulating hormone (TSH)
- ❑ Arrange for follow-up visit
- ❑ Verbal contracting with patient to call or seek immediate help if any suicidal ideation develops

Total Score: _____ / 29

Passing score for this station is 20 correct items.

Communication and Interpersonal Skills (CIS) Scoresheet

Please rate each of the following items on a scale from 1–10.
These items may be completed by either the standardized patient or another student.

Scoresheet 1

	Poor		Fair		Good		Very Good		Excellent	
Professional appearance	1	2	3	4	5	6	7	8	9	10
Introduces self and shakes hands	1	2	3	4	5	6	7	8	9	10
Nonverbal communication (eye contact, facial expressiveness, body language)	1	2	3	4	5	6	7	8	9	10
Communicates effectively (open-ended questions, avoids jargon)	1	2	3	4	5	6	7	8	9	10
Establishes rapport with patient (empathy, appears nonjudgmental)	1	2	3	4	5	6	7	8	9	10
Allows patient to speak without being interrupted	1	2	3	4	5	6	7	8	9	10
Listens and seems to understand patient's concerns	1	2	3	4	5	6	7	8	9	10
Overall professionalism	1	2	3	4	5	6	7	8	9	10

Total Score:

Passing score for CIS section is 56 points.

Spoken English Proficiency (SEP) Scoresheet

Please rate each of the following items on a scale from 1–10.
These items may be completed by either the standardized patient or another student.

Scoresheet 2

	Poor		Fair		Good		Very Good		Excellent	
Examiner is articulate and easily understood	1	2	3	4	5	6	7	8	9	10
Pronunciation (words pronounced correctly; accent does not hinder communication)	1	2	3	4	5	6	7	8	9	10
Word choice is appropriate	1	2	3	4	5	6	7	8	9	10
Ability to communicate without excessive listener effort required to understand questions or responses	1	2	3	4	5	6	7	8	9	10
Patient's ability to understand the examiner	1	2	3	4	5	6	7	8	9	10
Examiner's ability to understand the patient	1	2	3	4	5	6	7	8	9	10

Total Score:

Passing score for SEP section is 42 points.

Diagnosis and Management of Depressive Illness

Overview

Depression is a very common disorder seen by primary care and sub-specialists alike. Depression may present as a primary illness as well as a common complication of almost all chronic diseases. It is common for patients to view depression as a "mental" problem rather than an organic disease or syndrome. Our increasing knowledge in the field of behavioral science and psychiatry indicates that a biological model may be used to describe and treat depression. When treating a depressed individual, it is helpful for that person to understand that depression is a legitimate illness with physical manifestations and that current treatments are often very effective in improving quality of life and overall function.

Recognizing Depression

Depression as a clinical syndrome is more than a disturbance of mood alone. The term "depressed" describes the feeling of sadness or feeling down. However, clinical depression is a more complex combination of symptoms leading to functional impairment in social, occupational, and marital arenas.

Medical students and house officers often find the mnemonic "**SIGE CAPS**" very helpful in screening for depression. To diagnose depression, there should be depressed mood and/or anhedonia *plus* at least four of the following for at least two weeks:

S—Sleep disturbance. Most commonly insomnia: difficulty falling asleep or maintaining restful sleep. Early morning awakening is a common symptom in depression.

I—Interests decreased (anhedonia). Not finding enjoyment in activities that were previously enjoyable. Patients may complain of excessive boredom, and may become more socially isolated.

G—Guilt. Nonspecific or recurring feelings of guilt. Other feelings of worthlessness or low self-esteem are also common.

E—Energy decreased. A common feature is fatigue or feeling excessively tired.

C—Concentration decreased. Patients often describe feeling mentally foggy or cloudy. Memory, especially short-term memory, may be impaired. Managing complex or multiple tasks may become difficult.

A—Appetite changes. This may be widely varied. Increased appetite and weight gain or decreased appetite and weight loss may be present.

P—Psychomotor changes. Agitation, feeling restless, sped up may be the dominant feature, or the patient may feel that he or she has slowed down and is moving or thinking in slow motion.

S—Suicidal ideation. All patients with the potential diagnosis of depression should be screened for this. Important questions include "Do you feel hopeless?" "Do you have thoughts of hurting yourself?" If a patient does have suicidal ideation, a more detailed history should be taken. Lethality assessment should include the level of detail and pre-planning regarding suicide. In addition, it should be asked if the patient has any availability of weapons, as they may be used in a suicide attempt.

Subtypes of Depressive Illness

Unipolar depression refers to depressed mood without manic features (see box on p. 114). Most general discussions of depression refer to this subtype.

Dysthymia is a chronic condition that may involve concurrent major depression or may exist as a low-grade state of melancholy for months to years. Dysthymia may be a lifelong condition and is often refractory to treatment.

Secondary depression refers to depressive symptoms caused by medication, drugs of abuse, or medical conditions. Symptoms may be mild or may result in major depression.

Premenstrual dysmorphic disorder includes a constellation of symptoms such as depressed mood, irritability, mood lability, headache (especially migraine), breast tenderness, edema, fatigue, and sleep difficulty that occur prior to menses. Symptoms interfere with work or social functioning and may become quite disabling.

Seasonal affective disorder refers to recurrent depression that occurs in annual cycles. Mood disturbance is linked to circadian rhythm disturbances caused by decreased sunlight exposure. It is most often seen in winter months, particularly in the Northern Hemisphere.

Postpartum depression occurs within weeks to months following delivery.

Bipolar disorder is characterized by the presence of mania, but may include depression. Recognition of bipolar disorder is important because its treatment may be much different than that of depression. In fact, medications used to treat unipolar depression may severely exacerbate manic symptoms and even precipitate overt psychosis. Like SIGE CAPS in depression, bipolar disorder also has a useful mnemonic, **DIG FAST** (see box on p. 114).

Depression with psychotic features and schizoaffective disorder refers to depression with concurrent hallucinations, delusions, or other psychotic behavior.

> **"DIG FAST" Mnemonic (Bipolar Disorder)**
>
> D—distractibility
> I—insomnia due to increased energy
> G—grandiosity
> F—flight of ideas, racing thoughts
> A—activity increased
> S—speech fast, excessive, or pressured
> T—thoughtlessness, impulsivity, recklessness, sexual promiscuity

Medical Evaluation

Because there are numerous medical conditions that may cause or precipitate depression, it is very important to take a complete medical history and review the medications of any patient suspected of having depression. The social history may reveal alcohol or drug abuse. A family history of psychiatric illness may help support the diagnosis.

Screening labs should include a CBC, TSH, and random blood glucose. Anemia, hyperthyroidism, hypothyroidism, and diabetes commonly present with depressive symptoms. Though conditions such as porphyria, syphilis, Wilson disease, and pancreatic cancer may present with depression, they are much less common and do not warrant screening in all cases of depression.

Treatment of Depression

Once the diagnosis of depression has been established, there are several modalities used to treat the patient. The decision of which combination to use should be made on a case-by-case basis.

Factors that influence the method of treatment include:

1. The degree of impairment
2. Duration of symptoms
3. Success or failure of prior treatments
4. The patient's perception of the disease
5. The patient's preference for each treatment option
6. The level of comfort on the clinician's part with the various modalities

Counseling and Psychotherapy

There are numerous forms of therapy that do not necessarily involve the use of medications. Counseling with a well-trained provider can be very beneficial in helping patients recover from a depressive episode. Mild to moderate depression is often triggered by a traumatic or stressful event. Providing patients with insight into the role of their stressors and their depression has been shown to be a therapeutic intervention.

Exercise

The role of regular physical activity is often overlooked, and there is a paucity of randomized controlled trials examining exercise in the treatment of depression. However, many patients find a significant reduction in their disease after only a few weeks of regular exercise, and several smaller studies support this idea.

Pharmacologic Treatment

Medications are a very important treatment modality, especially in moderate to severe cases. There are numerous randomized controlled studies to support their efficacy, though there is not a great deal of evidence to show that one class of medication is any more effective than any other. The safety and side-effect profile, however, indicates that the selective serotonin reuptake inhibitors (SSRIs) generally may be more favorable. However, each patient needs to be considered individually in determining which medication may be best suited.

SSRIs

More recently, the selective serotonin reuptake inhibitors (SSRIs) have gained extremely wide and common use in the treatment of depression. In general, as a class these medications are quite safe and effective when used at appropriate dosages and for an adequate duration. Examples include fluoxetine (10 to 80 mg daily), sertraline (50 to 200 mg daily), and paroxetine (10 to 60 mg daily), though there are numerous others. Extreme caution and possibly avoidance of this class of medications should be exercised when treating children and adolescents due to the increased risk of suicide among these patients while on these medications.

Tricyclic/Heterocyclic Antidepressants

As an older class of medications, this group is less often used as monotherapy in the treatment of depression. There are numerous potential side effects to be aware of, including the risk of fatal overdose. The anticholinergic and antihistaminic/sedative effects vary widely within this class with amitriptyline being the most anticholinergic and sedating and desipramine being the least. More recently, this class of medications has gained wide use in the treatment of myofascial pain, chronic pain syndromes, peripheral neuropathy, and headache prophylaxis.

Newer Antidepressants

Several newer antidepressants have been developed in recent years that have less specific activity than the SSRIs. Some have norepinephrine reuptake inhibiting properties (such as venlafaxine) while others have dopamine and norepinephrine receptor affinity (such as bupropion).

Monoamine Oxidase Inhibitors (MAOIs)

MAOIs represent a much older and less commonly used class of antidepressants. MAOIs have significant side effects and, more important, potentially fatal drug–drug interactions. As such, they are not used very often anymore. In rare cases, a specialist may use MAOIs to treat refractory depression.

Other Treatment Options

Light Therapy: Light therapy has been shown to be both safe and effective in the treatment of seasonal affective disorder, particularly in mild to moderate cases.

Electroconvulsive Therapy: Like several other early breakthroughs in psychiatry and neurology, electroconvulsive therapy was discovered through serendipity. It was noted that patients with depression who suffered seizures had an improvement in their depressive symptoms. Seizures were then induced by iatrogenic hypoglycemia or transcranial electrocution (the former is no longer used due to significant patient risk). Although the seizures do decrease depressive symptoms, there are significant risks and side effects, including amnesia. Since the advent of more refined pharmaceuticals, electroconvulsive therapy is only seldom utilized, though it may be useful in some cases of refractory depression.

REFERENCES

American Psychiatric Association. Task Force on DSM-IV. Diagnostic and Statistical Manual of Mental Disorders: DSM-IV, 4th ed. Washington, DC, American Psychiatric Association, 1994.

Bhatia SC, Bhatia SK. Major depression: Selecting safe and effective treatment. Am Fam Physician 1997;55:1683–1694.

Boswell EB, Stoudemire A. Major depression in the primary care setting. Am J Med 1996;101:35–95.

Cole JO; Bodkin JA. Antidepressant side effects. J Clin Psychiatry 1990;51(1):21–26.

Esposito K; Goodnick P. Predictors of response in depression. Psychiatr Clin North Am 2003;26(2): 353–365.

Gold LH. Postpartum disorders in primary care: Diagnosis and treatment. Primary Care 2002;29:27–41.

Hirschfeld RMA, Clayton PJ, Cohen I, et al. Practice guideline for the treatment of patients with bipolar disorder. Am J Psychiatry 1994;151:1–31.

Keck PE Jr, McElroy SL, Arnold LM. Bipolar disorder. Med Clin North Am 2001;85(3):645–661.

Nierenberg AA, Wright EC. Evolution of remission as the new standard in the treatment of depression. J Clin Psychiatry 1999;60(S22):7–11.

Nobler MS, Sackheim HA. Electroconvulsive therapy: Clinical and biological aspects. In: Goodnick PJ, ed. Predictors of Treatment Response in Mood Disorders. Washington, DC, American Psychiatric Press, 1996, pp 177–198.

Parker G, Roy K, Wilhelm K, et al. Assessing the comparative effectiveness of antidepressant therapies: A prospective clinical practice study. J Clin Psychiatry 2001;62:117–125.

Partonen T, Lonnqvist J. Seasonal affective disorder. Lancet 1998;352:1369–1374.

Regier DA, Farmer ME, Rae DS, et al. Comorbidity of mental disorders with alcohol and other drug abuse: Results from the Epidemiologic Catchment Area Study. JAMA 1990;264:2511–2518.

Steiner M, Born L. Diagnosis and treatment of premenstrual dysphoric disorder: An update. Int Clin Psychopharmacol 2000;15(suppl 3):S5–S17.

Tollefson GD. Antidepressant treatment and side effect considerations. J Clin Psychiatry 1991;52(5-suppl): 4–13.

Wells BG, Mandos LA, Hayes PE. Depressive disorders. In: Pharmacotherapy: A Pathophysiologic Approach, 3rd ed. 1996. Stamford, CT: Appleton & Lange.

"I Keep Coughing"

Examinee Prompt

You are seeing this 31-year-old patient in an outpatient clinic for a chief complaint of "cough." Please complete the following tasks:

- Obtain a complete yet focused history
- Perform an appropriate physical examination.

You have 15 minutes to complete your visit with the patient. When you have finished your interaction with the patient, you may leave the examination room. Following your visit with the patient, you will be asked to write a complete progress note in the SOAP (Subjective, Objective, Assessment and Plan) format. You will have 10 additional minutes to complete the progress note.

Vital Signs

Temperature .... 102.6°F by oral measurement

Heart rate 104

Blood pressure 124/86

Respiratory rate 18

Room air pulse oximetry 96%

Patient Prompt

Background: You are seeing a doctor in the emergency department for an acute illness. You may offer any of the following information if specifically asked.

Chief Complaint: Cough and fever

History of the Present Illness: 31-year-old patient with a complaint of cough and fever. The illness began 5 days ago with what seemed to be a typical "cold." The symptoms began with a mild sore throat and clear rhinorrhea. Over the last 3 days, you have developed a worsening cough productive of dark yellow sputum (on one occasion your cough produced rusty, blood-streaked phlegm). You have had fevers for the last 2 days where you felt very hot but no temperature was recorded. You have also had chills but no rigors. You deny shortness of breath at rest, but do have dyspnea with mild to moderate physical exertion, which is unusual for you. You missed work for the last 4 days due to malaise, which is also very atypical.

Past Medical History:

- Otherwise healthy
- No history of asthma or chronic lung disease
- No history of cardiac disease

Past Surgical History: None

Medications:

- Tylenol 650 mg four times per day for fevers
- Robitussin DM (over the counter)
- Vitamin C 1500 mg lozenges 2 to 3 per day
- No recent use of antibiotics

Allergies: No known drug allergies

Social History:

- Single
- You work at a copy center
- Recently engaged
- No tobacco
- Approximately two beers per week
- No recent travel
- No pets

Family History: Parents and siblings are all healthy.

Review of Systems: No chest pain, no mental status changes, no headaches, no rashes, no arthralgias. Decreased oral intake but no nausea or vomiting. Normal urination.

Additional Information: During the pulmonary exam, please state "the pulmonary exam reveals rales in the right mid-lung field with scattered rhonchi but no wheezes. Air movement is good."

Pneumonia Scoresheet

Subjective

- ❑ Asks chief complaint
- ❑ Asks about fever and chills
- ❑ Duration of symptoms
- ❑ Asks about shortness of breath
- ❑ Asks about chest pain
- ❑ Asks about sputum production
- ❑ Malaise
- ❑ Past medical history (in particular no history of cardiac or pulmonary disease)
- ❑ Allergies
- ❑ Medications
- ❑ Asks about tobacco use
- ❑ Asks about alcohol use
- ❑ Travel history
- ❑ Animal exposure

Objective

- ❑ General appearance
- ❑ Cardiovascular exam
- ❑ Auscultation of the lungs
- ❑ Percussion of the lungs

Assessment (The following diagnosis should appear in the differential diagnosis)

- ❑ Community-acquired pneumonia

Plan

- ❑ Chest x-ray
- ❑ Complete blood count (CBC)
- ❑ Chemistry panel (electrolytes, blood urea nitrogen [BUN], creatinine, glucose)
- ❑ Pulse oximetry or arterial blood gas

Total Score: _____ / 23

Passing score for this station is 16 correct items.

Communication and Interpersonal Skills (CIS) Scoresheet

Please rate each of the following items on a scale from 1–10.
These items may be completed by either the standardized patient or another student.

Scoresheet 1

	Poor		Fair		Good		Very Good		Excellent	
Professional appearance	1	2	3	4	5	6	7	8	9	10
Introduces self and shakes hands	1	2	3	4	5	6	7	8	9	10
Nonverbal communication (eye contact, facial expressiveness, body language)	1	2	3	4	5	6	7	8	9	10
Communicates effectively (open-ended questions, avoids jargon)	1	2	3	4	5	6	7	8	9	10
Establishes rapport with patient (empathy, appears nonjudgmental)	1	2	3	4	5	6	7	8	9	10
Allows patient to speak without being interrupted	1	2	3	4	5	6	7	8	9	10
Listens and seems to understand patient's concerns	1	2	3	4	5	6	7	8	9	10
Overall professionalism	1	2	3	4	5	6	7	8	9	10

Total Score:

Passing score for CIS section is 56 points.

Spoken English Proficiency (SEP) Scoresheet

Please rate each of the following items on a scale from 1–10.
These items may be completed by either the standardized patient or another student.

Scoresheet 2

	Poor		Fair		Good		Very Good		Excellent	
Examiner is articulate and easily understood	1	2	3	4	5	6	7	8	9	10
Pronunciation (words pronounced correctly; accent does not hinder communication)	1	2	3	4	5	6	7	8	9	10
Word choice is appropriate	1	2	3	4	5	6	7	8	9	10
Ability to communicate without excessive listener effort required to understand questions or responses	1	2	3	4	5	6	7	8	9	10
Patient's ability to understand the examiner	1	2	3	4	5	6	7	8	9	10
Examiner's ability to understand the patient	1	2	3	4	5	6	7	8	9	10

Total Score:

Passing score for SEP section is 42 points.

Approach to the Patient With Community-Acquired Pneumonia

Overview

Bacterial pneumonia is a common condition that is potentially life-threatening, particularly in older adults and in those with underlying illnesses. Community-acquired pneumonia is the sixth leading cause of death in the United States, and the number one cause of death from infectious disease. There are numerous guidelines that may help a clinician in the decision-making process in the patient with pneumonia or suspected pneumonia. However, if one has a thorough understanding of the pathogenesis, antimicrobial profiles, and treatments for pneumonia, much of the decision making becomes an art of medicine issue. You should feel comfortable with the standard workup and rational therapeutics for pneumonia rather than relying on treatment algorithms. The following discussion provides this necessary information.

Diagnosing Pneumonia

The diagnosis of pneumonia begins with a clinical suspicion, which is a point that cannot be overstated. Though many patients may present with classic signs and symptoms such as productive cough, fever, malaise, and abnormal breath sounds and crackles on physical examination, many cases of pneumonia present in a more indolent or challenging manner. Younger patients may appear clinically well and have symptoms more consistent with a viral syndrome. Conversely, older patients or those with an inadequate immune response may present with nonrespiratory symptoms such as falling down, confusion, failure to thrive, or worsening of an underlying chronic illness.

When pneumonia is suspected, posteroanterior and lateral chest radiographs are recommended, not only to establish the diagnosis, but also to suggest other specific etiologies or conditions such as lung abscess, tuberculosis, or multilobar pneumonia. Sputum Gram stain and culture are included in some treatment algorithms, but are somewhat controversial. It is unclear if obtaining sputum is warranted in the outpatient setting. Sputum Gram stain and culture often are performed if the patient's disease is significant enough to warrant hospitalization. However, starting therapy in a timely manner is more important than determining a specific etiology, so if obtaining sputum sample will delay treatment, it does not need to be performed.

Testing for *Legionella* with a urinary antigen should be performed in cases of severe community-acquired pneumonia or if the patient fails to respond to initial treatment. Likewise, tuberculosis should be considered if a patient fails to respond to initial therapy or if the clinical scenario is suspicious for tuberculosis. A CBC is often helpful for assessing the severity of illness.

Etiology

The management of community-acquired pneumonia has changed over the past decade due to the identification of new pathogens, new methods of diagnosis, the availability of new antibiotics, and emerging resistance patterns. The clinician should be aware of the likely etiology of community-acquired pneumonia in different settings. Table 1 provides a list of pathogens involved in community-acquired pneumonia. This list is not exhaustive but provides the more common etiologic organisms.

When to Admit?

There are numerous published guidelines that attempt to answer this question of which patients require hospital admission. Unfortunately, many of the prognostic scoring tools were designed to predict mortality from pneumonia, not to determine which patients would need hospital admission. When any of the prognostic scoring tools are utilized, they should be used as adjunctive tools to support, not to replace, the clinical decision-making process. The decision of which patients to admit is an "art of medicine" decision that should be based on sound clinical judgment.

In some instances, it is quite clear that a patient should be hospitalized. For example, a patient with hypoxemia, the patient with multiple cardiopulmonary comorbidities, and the patient with impending respiratory failure clearly should all be admitted. However, in many cases the correct decision is not as clear. The decision to treat an individual as an outpatient should be done with caution and sound reasoning. The following factors should be included in this decision making:

- Age of patient (older patients are at higher risk, particularly beyond age 50)
- Coexisting cardiopulmonary disease or multiple medical conditions
- Tachycardia (heart rate >120)
- Tachypnea (respiratory rate >30)
- Significant dyspnea and/or hypoxia (Sao_2 <93% on room air)
- Temperature >38.5°C. Hypothermia (temperature <35°C is also worrisome)

Table 1

Pathogens Associated with Community-Acquired Pneumonia

Common Pathogens
Streptococcus pneumoniae
Haemophilus influenzae
Mycoplasma pneumoniae
Chlamydia pneumoniae
Moraxella catarrhalis
Legionella pneumoniae
Anaerobes
Mixed infection (bacteria plus an atypical pathogen or virus)
Less Common Pathogens
Enteric Gram negatives
Staphylococcus aureus
Mycobacterium tuberculosis
Neisseria meningitides
Streptococcus pyogenes
Pneumocystis carinii
Respiratory viruses
Endemic fungi

- Leukocytosis (WBC >14,000), bandemia, or leukopenia
- Oliguria
- Hypotension (serial blood pressure <90)
- Any mental status changes
- End-organ failure (e.g., elevated creatinine)
- Immunocompromised patient (diabetes, AIDS, chronic steroid use)
- Alcoholism
- Malnutrition
- Bilateral or multilobar infiltrates
- Electrolyte abnormalities (acidosis, hyponatremia, elevated BUN)
- Recent use of antibiotics

Patient Stratification

Patients may also be stratified based on underlying comorbidities to help determine which organisms are more likely to be the etiologic agent as well as to help guide the choice of antibiotic. This idea of patient stratification is supported by the American Thoracic Society in their management guidelines for community-acquired pneumonia.

Patients are first stratified based on coexisting cardiopulmonary disease, particularly chronic obstructive pulmonary disease (COPD) and congestive heart failure (CHF). Modifying risk factors that increase the risk of infection with specific pathogens are then considered. These modifying factors increase the risk of drug-resistant pneumococci (DRSP), enteric gram-negatives, and *Pseudomonas aeruginosa*. On the basis of these factors, patients are stratified into one of four groups, which are used to guide selection of appropriate therapy.

The following factors increase the risk of DRSP as an etiologic agent:

- Age >65 years
- Beta-lactam therapy within the past 3 months
- Alcoholism
- Immune-suppressive illness, including therapy with corticosteroids
- Multiple medical comorbidities
- Exposure to a child in a day care center

The following factors increase the risk of enteric gram-negatives as an etiologic agent:

- Residence in a nursing home
- Underlying cardiopulmonary disease
- Multiple medical comorbidities
- Recent antibiotic therapy

The following factors increase the risk of *Pseudomonas aeruginosa* as an etiologic agent:

- Structural lung disease (bronchiectasis)
- Corticosteroid therapy at more than 10 mg per day
- Broad-spectrum antibiotic therapy for more than 7 days in the past month
- Malnutrition

Once underlying cardiopulmonary disease (COPD and CHF) and the modifying risk factors have been considered, patients can be stratified into one of four groups for the purposes of guiding antimicrobial choices.

Group 1: Outpatient, no cardiopulmonary disease, no modifying risk factors

Group 2: Outpatient with cardiopulmonary disease and/or other modifying risk factors

Group 3: Inpatient, not in intensive care unit (ICU)

Group 4: Patients admitted to ICU

Antibiotic Selection

The following suggested therapies conform to American Thoracic Society guidelines. Please be aware that other guidelines exist, such as those published by the Centers for Disease Control, the Infectious Disease Society of American, and the Canadian Community Acquired Pneumonia recommendations.

Group 1: Outpatient, no cardiopulmonary disease, no modifying risk factors
Advanced generation macrolide (azithromycin or clarithromycin)

or

Doxycycline

Group 2: Outpatient, with cardiopulmonary disease and/or other modifying risk factors
Beta-lactam *plus* a macrolide or doxycycline

or

Antipneumococcal fluoroquinolone used alone (levofloxacin, sparfloxacin, moxifloxacin, gatifloxacin)

Group 3: Inpatient, not in ICU
Intravenous ß-lactam *plus* IV or oral macrolide or doxycycline

or

Monotherapy with an antipneumococcal fluoroquinolone

Group 4: Patients admitted to ICU with no risks for *Pseudomonas aeruginosa*
IV ß-lactam

plus either

IV azithromycin or IV fluoroquinolone

Group 4: Patients admitted to ICU with risks for *Pseudomonas aeruginosa*
Selected IV antipseudomonal ß-lactam plus IV antipseudomonal quinolone (ciprofloxacin)

or

IV antipseudomonal ß-lactam plus IV aminoglycoside

plus either

IV azithromycin or IV nonpseudomonal fluoroquinolone

Clinical Response

Most patients with community-acquired pneumonia will have an adequate clinical response within 3 days of starting antimicrobial therapy. If the patient does not improve as expected, the initial diagnosis as well as host and pathogen factors should be reevaluated. Additionally, a search for complications of pneumonia such as empyema or lung abscess should be considered.

REFERENCES

Atlas SJ, Benzer TI, Borowsky LH, et al. Safely increasing the proportion of patients with community-acquired pneumonia treated as outpatients: An interventional trial. Arch Intern Med 1998;158:1350–1356.

Bernstein JM.Treatment of community-acquired pneumonia—IDSA guidelines. Infectious Diseases Society of America. Chest 1999;115(3 suppl):9S–13S.

Fang GD, Fine M, Orloff J, et al. New and emerging etiologies for community-acquired pneumonia with implication for therapy: A prospective multicenter study of 359 cases. Medicine 1990;69:307–316.

Fine MJ, Auble TE, Yealy DM, et al. A prediction rule to identify low-risk patients with community-acquired pneumonia. N Engl J Med 1997;336:243–250.

Fine MJ, Smith MA, Carson CA. Prognosis and outcomes of patients with community-acquired pneumonia: A meta-analysis. JAMA 1996;275:134–141.

Metlay JP, Fine MJ. Testing strategies in the initial management of patients with community-acquired pneumonia. Ann Intern Med 2003;138(2):109–118.

Niederman MS, Mandell LA, Anzueto A, et al. Guidelines for the management of adults with community-acquired pneumonia. Diagnosis, assessment of severity, antimicrobial therapy, and prevention. Am J Respir Crit Care Med 2001;163(7):1730–1754.

Porath A, Schlaeffer F, Lieberman D. Appropriateness of hospitalization of patients with community-acquired pneumonia. Ann Emerg Med 1996;27:176–183.

"My Pressures Definitely Are High"

Examinee Prompt

You are working in your primary care office and are seeing this 38-year-old male patient, who is a new patient to you, for a follow-up visit from urgent care. Please perform the following tasks:

- Obtain a focused history relevant to the patient's medical condition
- Perform an appropriate physical examination

Following your visit with this patient, please write a complete progress note using the standard SOAP (Subjective, Objective, Assessment and Plan) format. You are *not* expected to discuss your diagnosis and plan with the patient model in this case, but if you have certain recommendations that you would make, this should be included in your progress note.

When you have all of the information that you need you may leave the exam room. You will have 15 minutes to complete the history and physical portion of this station and 10 additional minutes to complete your progress note.

Vital Signs

Temperature .... 98.6°F

Blood pressure left arm 152/96

Blood pressure right arm 149/99

Heart rate .... 80 (regular)

Respiratory rate 14

Patient Prompt

Background: You are a 38-year-old male patient seeing your newly assigned physician. You were seen in an urgent care clinic 3 weeks ago for conjunctivitis, and your blood pressure was noted to be elevated. The doctor in urgent care asked you to check your blood pressures at home and follow up with your primary care physician. You have kept an extensive record of your home blood pressure measurements.

Chief Complaint: Blood pressure check

History of the Present Illness: 38-year-old patient seen in urgent care 3 weeks ago for a diagnosis of acute infectious conjunctivitis, which has since resolved. Incidentally, an elevated blood pressure was noted and confirmed. You have kept a record of your home blood pressure measurements as requested. You are completely asymptomatic. If asked, you may provide the record of blood pressure measurements on the following page to the examiner. Though you have not been diagnosed with high blood pressure in the past, you have not seen a medical provider for more than 15 years.

Past Medical and Surgical History: Obsessive compulsive disorder, untreated

Medications: None

Allergies: No known drug allergies

Family History: Father and two brothers have been diagnosed with high blood pressure. You do not know of any other family medical history, including diabetes or coronary artery disease.

Social History:
- You work at a data entry service
- You are single and not sexually active
- You do not smoke or drink alcohol
- Your diet consists mainly of fast food (two meals per day)
- You do not exercise at all

Review of Systems:
- No headaches, sweating, palpitations, or blurry vision
- No chest pain, shortness of breath, orthopnea, paroxysmal nocturnal dyspnea, dyspnea on exertion
- No erectile dysfunction or claudication
- No history of loud snoring or excessive daytime somnolence
- Review of systems is otherwise completely negative

Additional Information: Your physical exam is completely normal other than elevated blood pressure.

Please provide the blood pressure log on the following page to the examiner.

My Blood Pressure Log

Urgent Care (10/17): 168/101, rechecked 159/99, rechecked 161/98.

Drug store (10/18): 156/94, rechecked 166/99, rechecked 170/90, rechecked 163/91, rechecked 160/92.

Health Fair at work (10/25): 149/89, rechecked 150/92—*They wouldn't let me check it again*!!

Drug store (later that day on 10/25) 149/92, 151/65, "error"—*I think I moved during this one*, 160/94, *was asked to let someone else use the machine*

Home blood pressure monitor:

10/26: 147/89

10/27: 151/96

10/29: 166/ 101

10/31: 160/95

11/2: 158/98

Hypertension Scoresheet

Subjective

- ❑ Asks chief complaint
- ❑ Confirm serial blood pressure measurements have been taken and recorded (needed to appropriately establish the diagnosis of hypertension)
- ❑ Asks about headaches, sweating, palpitations, or blurry vision (credit for asking any)
- ❑ Asks about chest pain, shortness of breath, orthopnea, paroxysmal nocturnal dyspnea, dyspnea on exertion (credit given for any cardiac symptom asked)
- ❑ Asks about erectile dysfunction or claudication (or other potential symptoms of peripheral vascular disease)
- ❑ Asks about history of loud snoring, excessive daytime somnolence
- ❑ Past medical history
- ❑ Medications
- ❑ Medication allergies
- ❑ Diet (including at least one of the following: sodium intake, caffeine, high fat)
- ❑ Drug use
- ❑ Use of over-the-counter stimulants or herbal stimulants
- ❑ Exercise habits
- ❑ Smoking
- ❑ Alcohol use
- ❑ Family history (credit given for any of the following: coronary artery disease, hypertension, diabetes, hyperlipidemia)

Objective

- ❑ Blood pressure measurements noted on progress note
- ❑ Optic fundi normal
- ❑ Thyroid gland is normal
- ❑ Cardiac examination normal
- ❑ Peripheral pulses normal
- ❑ No carotid or abdominal bruits (credit given for either)
- ❑ Jugular venous pulsations are normal (not elevated or distended)
- ❑ Lungs are clear
- ❑ Abdominal exam normal without mass or enlarged palpable aorta
- ❑ No lower extremity edema

Assessment

(the following item should be included in the differential diagnosis)

- ❑ Hypertension (uncomplicated)

Plan

- ❑ Dietary counseling (avoid excess sodium, alcohol, caffeine)
- ❑ Exercise counseling
- ❑ Home/ambulatory blood pressure monitoring (consider bringing machine to next visit to ensure machine is accurate)
- ❑ Return visit suggested (preferably 6 to 8 weeks)
- ❑ Laboratory data ordered (up to five points for the following answers):
  - ❍ Electrolytes
  - ❍ Serum blood urea nitrogen (BUN), creatinine
  - ❍ Serum calcium
  - ❍ Serum thyroid-stimulating hormone (TSH)
  - ❍ Fasting lipid profile
  - ❍ Random or fasting blood glucose
  - ❍ Urinalysis (or urine microalbumin)

Total Score: _____ / 36

Passing score for this station is 25 correct items.

Communication and Interpersonal Skills (CIS) Scoresheet

Please rate each of the following items on a scale from 1–10.
These items may be completed by either the standardized patient or another student.

Scoresheet 1

	Poor		Fair		Good		Very Good		Excellent	
Professional appearance	1	2	3	4	5	6	7	8	9	10
Introduces self and shakes hands	1	2	3	4	5	6	7	8	9	10
Nonverbal communication (eye contact, facial expressiveness, body language)	1	2	3	4	5	6	7	8	9	10
Communicates effectively (open-ended questions, avoids jargon)	1	2	3	4	5	6	7	8	9	10
Establishes rapport with patient (empathy, appears nonjudgmental)	1	2	3	4	5	6	7	8	9	10
Allows patient to speak without being interrupted	1	2	3	4	5	6	7	8	9	10
Listens and seems to understand patient's concerns	1	2	3	4	5	6	7	8	9	10
Overall professionalism	1	2	3	4	5	6	7	8	9	10

Total Score:

Passing score for CIS section is 56 points.

Spoken English Proficiency (SEP) Scoresheet

Please rate each of the following items on a scale from 1–10.
These items may be completed by either the standardized patient or another student.

Scoresheet 2

	Poor		Fair		Good		Very Good		Excellent	
Examiner is articulate and easily understood	1	2	3	4	5	6	7	8	9	10
Pronunciation (words pronounced correctly; accent does not hinder communication)	1	2	3	4	5	6	7	8	9	10
Word choice is appropriate	1	2	3	4	5	6	7	8	9	10
Ability to communicate without excessive listener effort required to understand questions or responses	1	2	3	4	5	6	7	8	9	10
Patient's ability to understand the examiner	1	2	3	4	5	6	7	8	9	10
Examiner's ability to understand the patient	1	2	3	4	5	6	7	8	9	10

Total Score:

Passing score for SEP section is 42 points.

Management of Arterial Hypertension

Overview

A review of the literature reveals a significant trend toward more aggressive management of hypertension. Although numerous studies support tight control of blood pressures, reality suggests that patients are not being treated according to current guidelines. While 50 million Americans have hypertension, it is well controlled in only one-third of these patients. With larger randomized controlled trials and an ever-increasing data pool, it is becoming clear that tighter control is vital to reducing morbidity and mortality due to heart disease, stroke, and end-organ damage. In light of the ALLHAT trial and the subsequent recommendations by JNC 7, the following discussion provides an overview of the current standard in managing hypertension.

Definitions

Any diagnosis of hypertension should be based upon two or more properly measured, seated blood pressure readings on each of two or more office visits, using an appropriate-sized cuff. The following reference points are provided by JNC 7:

- Normal adult blood pressure is <120/80.
- Elevated blood pressure or "pre-hypertension" is 120–139/80–89.
- Hypertension is >140/90 (or >130/80 in a patient with diabetes or renal disease)

Medical Evaluation of Newly Diagnosed Hypertension

Once the diagnosis of hypertension is established, secondary causes of hypertension should be ruled out. It is also important to evaluate a patient for end-organ complications that may have already occurred as a result of untreated or inadequately treated hypertension. The initial workup should include the following items:

- Blood pressure measurement in both arms
- Examination of the optic fundi
- Palpation of the thyroid gland
- Thorough cardiovascular exam (including pulses, palpation of the abdominal aorta, auscultation for carotid or abdominal bruits)
- Serum electrolytes, BUN, creatinine (to screen for kidney disease, Cushing syndrome, and mineralocorticoid excess)
- TSH, calcium (to screen for thyroid, and parathyroid disease)
- Urinalysis or urine microalbumin (to screen for microalbuminuria and proteinuria, which indicate kidney damage)
- 12-lead electrocardiogram (ECG) (to screen for left ventricular hypertrophy and prior ischemia, as well as to document a baseline)
- Blood glucose (to screen for diabetes or insulin resistance)
- CBC
- Fasting lipid profile

One should consider the following tests if the underlying disease is suspected as a cause of hypertension (though these are much less common and are not necessary for routine screening):

- Urine catecholamine screening (when pheochromocytoma is suspected)
- Urine drug screening (to screen for drugs of abuse)
- Chest computed tomography (CT). (In a young patient with hypertension, one should consider coarctation of the aorta. Blood pressure is typically higher in the upper limbs in comparison to the lower, and patients often have a murmur.)
- Sleep study (when sleep apnea is suspected). Sleep apnea classically presents with the triad of daytime somnolence, loud snoring, and hypertension.
- High sensitivity C-reactive protein and fasting homocysteine (may be indicated if there is a strong family history of early cardiovascular disease).
- Renal artery duplex, magnetic resonance imaging (MRI), renal scan, or serum renin level (when renal artery stenosis is suspected, particularly in young patients, those with refractory hypertension, or if there is a significant elevation of the serum creatinine while on an angiotensin-converting enzyme inhibitor).

Interventions and Treatments for Hypertension

For patients at risk for hypertension, or patients with newly diagnosed pre-hypertension, the following interventions have been shown to be effective in prevention or early treatment:

- Weight loss
- Restriction of sodium intake
- DASH diet (Dietary Approaches to Stop Hypertension)

- Moderation of alcohol use
- Regular cardiovascular exercise

Medications may be indicated if the patient is diagnosed with hypertension. There is recent evidence to suggest that thiazide diuretics are preferable as first-line agents, though treatment should be individualized to each patient. Some commonly used antihypertensive classes are outlined in Table 1.

Monotherapy vs. Combination of Agents?

As with any medical condition, it is always preferable to use the lowest dose and the fewest number of agents to achieve a therapeutic goal. In the treatment of hypertension, especially in moderate to severe cases, there is a significant body of evidence to suggest that patients are more likely to eventually require more than one medication. In an effort to achieve ideal control of blood pressures and minimize side effects, there currently is a trend to use more than one antihypertensive agent or use a combination agent, a strategy that is supported by the ACCOMPLISH trial.

Special Considerations

There are several conditions in which treatment options may be different from that of the "normal" uncomplicated hypertensive patient.

Known Coronary Artery Disease

Randomized controlled trials have shown ß-blockers and angiotensin-converting enzyme (ACE) inhibitors (or angiotensin receptor blockers, or ARBs) to be of significant benefit. In patients with chronic angina, in whom rate control is also important, calcium channel blockers are also useful.

Congestive Heart Failure

ACE inhibitors and diuretics (loop or thiazide) have been shown to be of benefit for both systolic and diastolic dysfunction. Although β-blockers were once thought to be contraindicated, they too are now commonly used because of their significant benefit. In cases of significant systolic dysfunction, aldosterone antagonists (spironolactone) have also gained favor due to their beneficial effects on mortality.

Table 1

Drug Class	Examples
Thiazide diuretics	Hydrochlorothiazide
Beta-blockers	Atenolol
	Propranolol
	Metoprolol
Angiotensin-converting enzyme inhibitors	Lisinopril
	Captopril
	Enalapril
Angiotensin II antagonists (Angiotensin receptor blockers)	Losartan
	Valsartan
Calcium channel blockers	Verapamil
	Diltiazem
	Amlodipine
	Nifedipine
Alpha-1 blockers	Prazosin
	Terazosin
Central alpha-2 agonists	Clonidine
Vasodilating agents	Hydralazine
Diuretics/other	Triamterene
	Spironolactone
	Lasix

Diabetes

Although any agent or combination of agents may be used to lower blood pressure in diabetes below the goal of <130/80, ACE inhibitors (or ARBs) have the additional benefit of preventing or delaying diabetic nephropathy.

Chronic Kidney Disease

As with diabetes, ACE inhibitors and ARBs commonly are used to protect against the progression of renal disease. As with diabetes, the goal blood pressure of <130/80 is also used. The caveat with patients with renal disease is that with increasing dosages, the potential risks of hyperkalemia and worsening azotemia should be noted and carefully monitored.

African-American Patients

Thiazide diuretics and calcium channel blockers may be more effective in this population as monotherapy, compared to ACE inhibitors and ß-blockers. However, in patients with microalbuminuria, proteinuria, or diabetes, an ACE inhibitor or ARB certainly should be strongly considered, especially in combination with a thiazide diuretic.

Elderly Patients

The elderly are both more likely to have hypertension and suffer from its complications. Nonpharmacologic interventions should be suggested for this population, at least initially, as these patients are also more prone to medication side effects. If, after close observation, these interventions are ineffective, medications may be indicated. It is reasonable to ask an elderly patient to stand while checking blood pressure as orthostasis can be a significant obstacle to medication tolerance and adherence. Low initial dosages and very slow titration of medication usually are required.

Benign Prostatic Hyperplasia (BPH)

Although diuretics are high on most treatment algorithms, the patient with BPH and urinary outlet obstructive symptoms potentially may be harmed by these mediations. In this case, the α_1 blockers are of particular benefit, as they may alleviate BPH symptoms and lower blood pressure.

Stroke

Hypertension is a major risk factor for stroke. Along with aggressive control of dyslipidemia and antiplatelet therapy, control of blood pressure is very important. Diuretics and ACE inhibitors are of particular benefit.

Pregnancy

ACE inhibitors and ARBs are contraindicated in pregnancy due to reported toxicity, especially in the second and third trimester; ß-blockers and methyldopa have more data to support their safety. Because intrauterine growth retardation has been reported in some patients taking atenolol, labetalol is often used when a beta-blocker is desired. Patients with preexisting chronic hypertension or newly diagnosed hypertension during pregnancy should be co-managed by a high-risk obstetrician.

REFERENCES

ACOG Practice Bulletin. Chronic hypertension in pregnancy. ACOG Committee on Practice Bulletins. Obstet Gynecol 2001;98:177–185.

Appel LJ, Champagne CM, Harsha DW, et al. Effects of comprehensive lifestyle modification on blood pressure control: Main results of the PREMIER clinical trial. Writing Group of the PREMIER Collaborative Research Group. JAMA 2003; 289:2083–2093.

Bakris GL, Williams M, Dworkin L, et al. Preserving renal function in adults with hypertension and diabetes: A consensus approach. National Kidney Foundation Hypertension and Diabetes Executive Committees Working Group. Am J Kidney Dis 2000; 36:646–661.

Chobanian AV, Bakris GL, Black HR, et al. The seventh report of the Joint National Committee on Prevention, Detection, Evaluation, and Treatment of High Blood Pressure: The JNC 7 report. JAMA 2003;289:2560–2572.

Cooper R, Rotimi C. Hypertension in blacks. Am J Hypertens 1997;10:804–812.

Devereux, RB, Ofili EO. A year since JNC 7: What's new about hypertension. Patient Care 2004;38:52–64.

Ebell MH. Initial evaluation of hypertension. Am Fam Physician 2004;69(6):1485–1487.

Ebell MH. A tool for evaluating hypertension. Fam Pract Manag 2004;11(3):79–81.

Expert Panel on Detection, Evaluation, and Treatment of High Blood Cholesterol in Adults. Third report of the National Cholesterol Education Program (NCEP) expert panel on detection, evaluation, and treatment of high blood cholesterol in adults (Adult Treatment Panel III): Final report. Circulation 2002;106:3143–3421.

Garg JP, Bakris GL. Microalbuminuria: Marker of vascular dysfunction, risk factor for cardiovascular disease. Vasc Med 2002;7:35–43.

Gregg AR. Hypertension in pregnancy. Obstet Gynecol Clin North Am 2004;31(2):223–241.

Hajjar I, Kotchen TA. Trends in prevalence, awareness, treatment, and control of hypertension in the United States, 1988–2000. JAMA 2003;290:199–206.

Hall WD. Resistant hypertension, secondary hypertension, and hypertensive crises. Cardiol Clin 2002; 20(2):281–289.

He J, Whelton PK, Appel LJ, Charleston J, Klag MJ. Long-term effects of weight loss and dietary sodium reduction on incidence of hypertension. Hypertension 2000;35:544–549.

Heart Outcomes Prevention Evaluation Study Investigators. Effects of an angiotensin-converting-enzyme inhibitor, ramipril, on cardiovascular events in high-risk patients. N Engl J Med 2000;342:145–153.

Jones DW, Appel LJ, Sheps SG, Roccella EJ, Lenfant C. Measuring blood pressure accurately: New and persistent challenges. JAMA 2003;289:1027–1030.

Kaplan NM. Management of hypertension in patients with type 2 diabetes mellitus: Guidelines based on current evidence. Ann Intern Med 2001;135:1079–1083.

Meissner I, Whisnant JP, Sheps SG, et al. Detection and control of high blood pressure in the community: Do we need a wake up call? Hypertension 1999;34:466–471.

O'Rorke JE, Richardson WS. Evidence-based management of hypertension: What to do when blood pressure is difficult to control. BMJ 2001;322:1229–1232.

Pickering TG. Principles and techniques of blood pressure measurement. Cardiol Clin 2002;20(2):207–223.

PROGRESS Collaborative Group. Randomised trial of a perindopril-based blood-pressure-lowering regimen among 6,105 individuals with previous stroke or transient ischaemic attack. Lancet 2001; 358:1033–1041.

Ridker PM, Rifai N, Rose L, Buring JE, Cook NR. Comparison of C-reactive protein and low-density lipoprotein cholesterol levels in the prediction of first cardiovascular events. N Engl J Med 2002;347: 1557–1565.

Ruzicka M, Leenen FH. Monotherapy versus combination therapy as first-line treatment of uncomplicated arterial hypertension. Drugs 2001;61:943–954.

Sacks FM, Svetkey LP, Vollmer WM, et al. Effects on blood pressure of reduced dietary sodium and the Dietary Approaches to Stop Hypertension (DASH) diet. DASH-Sodium Collaborative Research Group. N Engl J Med 2001;344:3–10.

Setaro JF, Black HR. Refractory hypertension. N Engl J Med 1992;327:543–547.

SHEP Cooperative Research Group. Prevention of stroke by antihypertensive drug treatment in older persons with isolated systolic hypertension. Final results of the Systolic Hypertension in the Elderly Program (SHEP). JAMA 1991;265:3255–3264.

The Acute Infarction Ramipril Efficacy (AIRE) Study Investigators. Effect of ramipril on mortality and morbidity of survivors of acute myocardial infarction with clinical evidence of heart failure. Lancet 1993;342:821–828.

The ALLHAT Officers and Coordinators for the ALLHAT Collaborative Research Group. Major outcomes in high-risk hypertensive patients randomized to angiotensin-converting enzyme inhibitor or calcium channel blocker vs. diuretic. The Antihypertensive and Lipid-Lowering Treatment to Prevent Heart Attack Trial (ALLHAT). JAMA 2002;288:2981–2997.

The SOLVD Investigators. Effect of enalapril on survival in patients with reduced left ventricular ejection fractions and congestive heart failure. N Engl J Med 1991;325:293–302.

UKPDS 39. Efficacy of atenolol and captopril in reducing risk of macrovascular and microvascular complications in type 2 diabetes: UKPDS 39. UK Prospective Diabetes Study Group. BMJ 1998;317:713–720.

U.S. Department of Health and Human Services, National Heart, Lung, and Blood Institute. National High Blood Pressure Education Program. Available at: http://www.nhlbi.nih.gov/about/nhbpep/index.htm. Accessed May 2005.

U.S. Preventive Services Task Force Screening for High Blood Pressure: Recommendations and rationale. Am Fam Physician 2003;68(10):2019–2022.

Vasan RS, Larson MG, Leip EP, et al. Impact of high-normal blood pressure on the risk of cardiovascular disease. N Engl J Med 2001;45:1291–1297.

Verdecchia P, Angeli F, Gattobigio R. Clinical usefulness of ambulatory blood pressure monitoring. J Am Soc Nephrol 2004;15(suppl 1):S30–S33.

Wilson PWF, D'Agostino RB, Parise H, Meigs JB. The metabolic syndrome as a precursor of cardiovascular disease and type 2 diabetes mellitus. Diabetes 2002; 51:A242.

Wofford MR, King DS, Wyatt SB, Jones DW. Secondary hypertension: Detection and management for the primary care provider. J Clin Hypertens 2000; 2:124–131.

"Can You Fix My Headaches?"

Examinee Prompt

You are seeing this 26-year-old man, who is a new patient to you, for a chief complaint of "headache." Please complete the following tasks:

- Obtain a focused history relevant to the patient's chief complaint.
- Perform an appropriate focused physical exam.
- Complete a progress note using the standard "SOAP" (Subjective, Objective, Assessment and Plan) format. For this station, please include treatment options in your plan.

Please discuss your diagnosis and treatment plan with the patient. When you have all of the information and have completed your discussion with the patient, you may leave the exam room. You will have 15 minutes to complete the history and physical portion of this station and 10 additional minutes to complete your progress note.

Patient Prompt

Background: You are a 26-year-old male patient complaining of intermittent headache for the past 2 years.

Chief Complaint: Headaches

History of the Present Illness: 26-year-old male patient with a 2-year history of intermittent headaches. The headaches occur once or twice per month. They pain is described as throbbing and ranges in intensity from 5 to 8/10 on a pain scale. The headaches usually begin unilaterally but often progress to become bilateral. They are associated with photophobia but no phonophobia. You sometimes become nauseated and have vomited on a few occasions. There has not been a significant change in the pattern of these headaches over the last 2 years. When the headaches occur, unusual lights are sometimes present in the usual visual fields. The headaches sometimes are relieved with ibuprofen, but often require sleeping in a dark, cool, quiet room for several hours to get complete relief. The headaches sometimes cause you to miss work or social functions. There is no change in the headaches with positional changes. They do not awake you from sleep. There is no history of head trauma.

Past Medical History: None

Past Surgical History: None

Medications: Ibuprofen as needed for headache

Allergies: No known drug allergies

Family History:

- Mother has had problems with headaches in the past, but you do not know much about them
- Father has hyperlipidemia

Social History:

- Engaged, no children
- Graduate student in business school
- No tobacco or drug use
- 2 to 3 beers per week
- Exercise 4 times per week

Review of Systems: Review of systems is completely negative except as noted in the history of the present illness. No fevers. No weakness, numbness, paresthesias, or dizziness. No changes in mental status, confusion, or difficulty with speech.

Additional Information: All physical exam findings are normal.

Headache Scoresheet

Subjective

- ❑ Asks chief complaint
- ❑ Location of pain
- ❑ Frequency
- ❑ Severity
- ❑ Aggravating/alleviating factors
- ❑ Nausea/vomiting
- ❑ Light/sound sensitivity
- ❑ Fevers
- ❑ Neurologic symptoms (credit for any of the following: numbness, weakness, difficulty with speech, mental status problems, visual changes)
- ❑ Frequency of symptoms
- ❑ Medications
- ❑ Past medical history
- ❑ History of trauma
- ❑ Social history (credit for any of the following: job, marital status, smoking, alcohol)

Objective

- ❑ Funduscopic exam
- ❑ Cranial nerves II through XII examined
- ❑ Palpation of scalp and neck for focal tenderness or reproduction of symptoms
- ❑ Evaluation for meningismus/neck stiffness
- ❑ Evaluation for gross sensory deficits
- ❑ Evaluation for gross motor deficits
- ❑ Assessment of gait

Diagnosis

- ❑ Correct diagnosis of migraine headache

Plan

- ❑ Discusses the option of prophylactic treatment (such as tricyclic antidepressants)
- ❑ Offers medical therapy beyond anti-inflammatory medications (such as a triptans)
- ❑ Plan does not include neuroimaging
- ❑ Indicates a follow-up plan

Total Score: _____ / 26

Passing score for this station is 18 correct items.

Communication and Interpersonal Skills (CIS) Scoresheet

Please rate each of the following items on a scale from 1–10.
These items may be completed by either the standardized patient or another student.

Scoresheet 1

	Poor		Fair		Good		Very Good		Excellent	
Professional appearance	1	2	3	4	5	6	7	8	9	10
Introduces self and shakes hands	1	2	3	4	5	6	7	8	9	10
Nonverbal communication (eye contact, facial expressiveness, body language)	1	2	3	4	5	6	7	8	9	10
Communicates effectively (open-ended questions, avoids jargon)	1	2	3	4	5	6	7	8	9	10
Establishes rapport with patient (empathy, appears nonjudgmental)	1	2	3	4	5	6	7	8	9	10
Allows patient to speak without being interrupted	1	2	3	4	5	6	7	8	9	10
Listens and seems to understand patient's concerns	1	2	3	4	5	6	7	8	9	10
Overall professionalism	1	2	3	4	5	6	7	8	9	10

Total Score:

Passing score for CIS section is 56 points.

Spoken English Proficiency (SEP) Scoresheet

Please rate each of the following items on a scale from 1–10.
These items may be completed by either the standardized patient or another student.

Scoresheet 2

	Poor		Fair		Good		Very Good		Excellent	
Examiner is articulate and easily understood	1	2	3	4	5	6	7	8	9	10
Pronunciation (words pronounced correctly; accent does not hinder communication)	1	2	3	4	5	6	7	8	9	10
Word choice is appropriate	1	2	3	4	5	6	7	8	9	10
Ability to communicate without excessive listener effort required to understand questions or responses	1	2	3	4	5	6	7	8	9	10
Patient's ability to understand the examiner	1	2	3	4	5	6	7	8	9	10
Examiner's ability to understand the patient	1	2	3	4	5	6	7	8	9	10

Total Score:

Passing score for SEP section is 42 points.

Standards for the Medical Care of the Adult Patient with Headache

Diagnosis

There are several important aspects to consider in the evaluation of the patient complaining of headache. As a priority, the clinician should consider the following:

1. Is there an acute emergency? Potentially worrisome features include the sudden onset of a severe headache (such as the so-called "thunderclap headache" indicating a subarachnoid hemorrhage), the presence of neurologic symptoms other than aura (such as weakness, numbness, paresthesias, speech difficulty, altered level of consciousness, ataxia, or seizure), the presence of focal or lateralizing neurologic deficits on exam, and associated constitutional symptoms such as fever, weight loss, or meningismus.
2. Is neuroimaging necessary? Although a patient's perception may differ, neuroimaging usually is not indicated. The majority of headache cases are indeed benign. Imaging is considered advisable for patients who have had any of the worrisome features mentioned in number one above. Neuroimaging may also be indicated for patients who have had a new significant change in their headache pattern, known history of malignancy, age >50, new onset or change in symptoms, recent head trauma, exertional or positional headaches, headache made worse by coughing or intercourse, or headache that awakens the patient from sleep. Immunocompromised patients and patients on anticoagulation also warrant special consideration.
3. Is specialty consultation appropriate? Some headache subtypes warrant assistance from a neurologist or headache specialist as the evaluation and management of certain headaches require more training and expertise. These subtypes include refractory headache, frequent headaches that fail to respond to prophylaxis (see below), complicated migraine, trigeminal neuralgia, cluster headache, or any worrisome headache. Though consultation is not required for these subtypes of headache, it may be considered.

Common Primary Headache Subtypes

Migraine

Presentation: Mnemonic "SULTANS"
This type of headache is often defined by:

1. *S*evere *U*ni*L*ateral *T*hrobbing pain made worse with physical *A*ctivity
2. Associated with *N*ausea and/or *S*ensitivity to light or sound (photophobia and phonophobia)

Headache with at least two features from number 1 above and one symptom from number 2 could be considered migraine if there is no reason to suspect an organic cause. The presence or absence of a preceding aura, usually consisting of visual disturbances or scotomata, does not in itself make the diagnosis or rule out the diagnosis. Migraines typically last 4 to 72 hours. Triggers include diet, emotional stress, menses, sleep deprivation, or changes in sleep patterns.

Treatment: The treatment of migraine can be divided into medications used to treat the acute headache (abortive) and agents used in their prevention (prophylaxis).

Abortive agents include nonsteroidal anti-inflammatory drugs (NSAIDs) such as naproxen or ibuprofen combined with an antiemetic such as metoclopramide or prochlorperazine.

Midrin and Cafergot have largely been replaced by the newer and more selective agents—the triptans.

Sumatriptan (Imitrex), rizatriptan (Maxalt), and naratriptan (Amerge) are a few examples of this rapidly expanding class of medications. Their pharmacokinetics/pharmacodynamics vary widely.

Dihydroergotamine (DHE) is also a valuable agent, especially to help abort a headache of prolonged duration.

Prophylactic agents include tricyclic antidepressants such as amitriptyline or nortriptyline, α-blockers, calcium channel blockers, and anticonvulsants.

Episodic Tension Type

Presentation: These headaches are also quite common. Tension-type headaches are often described as a pressure, ache, tightness, or "band-like constriction" around the head. The severity of these symptoms does not generally influence the diagnosis. A stressful event may precipitate these headaches, as can the resolution of a stressful experience (the so-called "let down headache"). The absence of headache on vacation or weekends suggests tension type. Location of symptoms is commonly cervical, occipital, or temporal, though numerous variants exist. Palpation of these areas may reveal tender points or trigger points that reproduce headache symptoms. Nausea with or without vomiting may be associated.

Previously these headaches were thought to be caused by actual muscle tension leading to pain. More recently, as our understanding of headache pathophysiology advances, this subset is thought to exist along a continuum with migraine. It is common for patients to suffer from both. A patient with a predominance of tension-type symptoms along with several migraine features may be described as having a "migrainous" headache.

Treatment: Treatment of tension-type headache is very similar to migraine in both abortive and prophylaxis with the exception of triptans, which are used only for migraine headaches.

Analgesic Rebound

Presentation: Analgesic rebound headache should be high on the differential for a patient with chronic daily headaches. Often a patient begins with migraine or tension-type headaches on an episodic basis. With frequent use of analgesics, either over the counter or prescribed, patients begin to require more medication (both in dose and frequency of use). These headaches are then thought to "transform" into analgesic rebound if not managed appropriately. Previously called "drug rebound" as it was thought that potent narcotics were to blame, these headaches actually may be caused by any agent. Combination medications such as Excedrin (caffeine, aspirin, and acetaminophen) are often implicated.

Treatment: The treatment of analgesic rebound must be focused on removing the offending agent. Many patients are often switched to a prophylactic agent for long-term management, using transitional medications during the "weaning" process. Discontinuation of the analgesic requires thorough communication by the physician and clear understanding by the patient regarding what is causing the headaches. Transitional medications include longer-acting NSAIDs (piroxicam, nabumetone), triptans (naratriptan, frovatriptan, etc.) and, in some cases, oral corticosteroids (Decadron).

Cluster Headache

Presentation: While much less common than the aforementioned types, cluster headaches may be quite incapacitating. These headaches often occur in attacks or clusters once or numerous times per day, with headache-free periods in between. Patients with cluster headaches often describe severe eye pain with associated lacrimation, redness, rhinorrhea, and nasal congestion.

Treatment: Medications sometimes used in the treatment of cluster headaches include indomethacin, methysergide, lithium carbonate, corticosteroids, sumatriptan, and DHE. Indomethacin is particularly effective in the treatment of chronic paroxysmal hemicrania, a subset of cluster headaches. Inhaled oxygen may also abort an acute attack. Prophylaxis may be achieved with various calcium channel blockers, divalproex, and topiramate, often in combination with the above abortive agents.

Trigeminal Neuralgia (Tic Douloureux)

Presentation: Like cluster headaches, trigeminal neuralgia usually causes unilateral headache or facial pain. The two are often confused. Patients usually describe rapid paroxysms of burning or lancinating pain along the distribution of the involved trigeminal nerve branch. Stimulation of the face by rubbing, chewing, talking, and so forth can evoke attacks.

Treatment: As these symptoms are often quite severe, most first-line low-potency analgesics are often ineffective. Anticonvulsants including carbamazepine, phenytoin, and gabapentin are commonly used therapeutic and/or prophylactic agents. Surgical or ablative treatment of the involved nerve branch should be considered for medication-refractory cases.

Secondary Headaches

Presentation: The list of potential sources of secondary headache is exhaustive. Brain tumor, subarachnoid hemorrhage, temporal arteritis, acute glaucoma, and acute bacterial meningitis should be considered, but their management would require interventions and treatment well beyond the scope of this exam. You should include these serious or potentially life-threatening conditions if asked to provide a differential diagnosis.

Key Physical Exam Points:
- Vital signs normal:
  - Fever may indicate an infectious or inflammatory process
  - Hypertension alone may cause headache but usually not until it is very high (systolic >200,

diastolic >110). Headaches associated with tachycardia make pheochromocytoma a consideration.

- Eye exam normal—including the funduscopic exam for papilledema (indicating increased intracranial pressure), no Horner syndrome, no gaze diplopia, and normal visual fields
- No temporal artery tenderness, swelling, or pulselessness
- Neck supple—no meningismus
- Neurologic exam normal—no gross focal or lateralizing deficits. This exam should include evaluation of cranial nerves, sensory, motor, station, and gait.

REFERENCES

Bernat JL, Vincent FM. Neurology: Problems in Primary Care, 2nd ed. Los Angeles, Practice Management Information Corporation, 1993, pp 131–163.

Blau JN, Thavapala M. Preventing migraine: A study of precipitating factors. Headache 1988;28: 481–483.

Capobianco DJ, Swanson JW, Dodick DW. Medication-induced (analgesic rebound) headache: Historical aspects and initial descriptions of the North American experience. Headache 2001;41(5):500–502.

Dodick D. Headache as a symptom of ominous disease. Postgrad Med 1997;101 (5):46–64.

Featherstone HJ. Migraine and muscle contraction headache: A continuum. Headache 1985;25: 194–198.

Headache Classification Committee of the International Headache Society. Classification and diagnostic criteria for headache disorders, cranial neuralgia, and facial pain. Cephalgia 1988;8(suppl 7):1–96.

Maizels M. The clinician's approach to the management of headache. West J Med 1998;168:203–212.

Spierings EL, Ranke AH, Honkoop PC. Precipitating and aggravating factors of migraine versus tension-type headache. Headache 2001;41:554–558.

“I’m Going Blind”

Examinee Prompt

You are seeing this 67-year-old female patient in your office for a chief complaint of "visual change in the right eye." Please complete the following tasks:

- Obtain a focused history relevant to this patient's complaint
- Conduct an appropriate physical examination

You have 15 minutes to complete your visit with the patient. When you have all of the information that you need you may leave the examination room. Following your visit with the patient, you will be asked to write a thorough progress note, including a suspected diagnosis and a treatment plan. You will have 10 additional minutes to complete the progress note.

For this case only, if consultation is desired, please make that part of your diagnostic and treatment plan.

Patient Prompt

Background: You are a 67-year-old patient who noticed flashing lights in the right eye this morning followed by large numbers of floaters. It then seemed that a shade obscured the vision in the right eye. You are understandably concerned about the visual loss.

Chief Complaint: Visual changes in the right eye

History of the Present Illness: 67-year-old patient who noticed flashing lights in the right eye this morning followed by large numbers of floaters. After the floaters appeared, it seemed that a shade obscured the vision in the right eye. The entire process occurred over an hour or two, and the vision loss has remained persistent. Vision in the left eye is completely normal. There is no pain in the eye, and you have not noticed any redness. There was no history of trauma to the eye. Vision has always been good, though you do use reading glasses. Looking at lights does not produce halos around the lights.

Past Medical History: Hypothyroidism

Past Surgical History: Hysterectomy at age 58 for uterine prolapse

Gynecologic History:
- As above. Last menstrual period age 48.
- Two normal spontaneous vaginal deliveries.

Medications:
- Levothyroxine 88 μg orally daily
- Aspirin 81 mg orally daily

Allergies: No known drug allergies

Family History:
- Both parents are in their late 80s and are healthy
- No family history of eye problems

Social History:
- Retired school teacher
- Married with two grown children
- No tobacco use
- One glass of wine with dinner

Review of Systems:
- No fever or chills
- No headaches
- No nausea or vomiting
- No extremity weakness or paresthesias
- Remainder of the review of systems is likewise negative

Additional Information:

- You have a friend who has a cataract and you ask the examiner if you could be suffering from a cataract.
- You also have a friend who is a bit older but who has macular degeneration. Please ask the examiner if this could be the cause of your vision loss.

Please familiarize yourself with the eye examination, as presented at the end of this chapter.

During the examination, if the examiner performs the following tests, or states that he or she would like to perform the tests, please provide him or her with the following information:

- External inspection: unremarkable
- Pupillary reaction testing: afferent papillary defect in the right eye
- Ocular mobility testing: normal
- For the purposes of this test, the examiner may ask to dilate the pupil. Please tell the examiner that pupillary dilation does not need to be performed on the standardized patient.
- Ophthalmoscopy: The retina appears elevated with folds.
- Intraocular pressure measurement: Please tell the examiner that this is normal if he or she mentions performing this test.
- Anterior chamber depth assessment: normal
- Confrontation field testing: intact bilaterally but blurry in the right eye
- Color vision testing: Materials are not available in the examination room for this test. Please tell the examiner that color vision testing is not required for the examination.
- Upper lid eversion: If the examiner wants to evert the upper lid, please state that the exam is unremarkable.
- Fluorescein staining: If the examiner wants to perform a fluorescein stain, please state that the exam is normal.

The examiner may ask about your visual acuity or ask if the nurse has performed a visual acuity examination. If the examiner asks about this or requests this information, you may provide the visual acuity measurements on the next page.

Visual Change Scoresheet

Subjective

- ❑ Baseline vision status
- ❑ Unilateral or bilateral vision loss
- ❑ History of trauma
- ❑ Timeline (abrupt or gradual onset)
- ❑ Eye pain
- ❑ Previous history of eye problems
- ❑ Past medical history
- ❑ Family history of eye problems

Objective

- ❑ Visual acuity noted
- ❑ External inspection of the eye and surrounding structures
- ❑ Pupillary reaction testing
- ❑ Ocular mobility testing
- ❑ Ophthalmoscopic examination
- ❑ Pupillary dilation performed before ophthalmoscopy
- ❑ Confrontation field testing

Assessment

- ❑ Suspected retinal detachment (this diagnosis should be included in the differential diagnosis)
- ❑ Credit for up to three of the items listed in the differential diagnosis of acute visual change in the text of this chapter
  - ❑ Diagnosis #1
  - ❑ Diagnosis #2
  - ❑ Diagnosis #3

Plan (these three items should be included in the plan)

- ❑ Visual acuity testing
- ❑ Slit-lamp examination
- ❑ Urgent ophthalmologic consultation

Total Score: ____ / 22

Passing score for this station is 15 correct items.

Communication and Interpersonal Skills (CIS) Scoresheet

Please rate each of the following items on a scale from 1–10.
These items may be completed by either the standardized patient or another student.

Scoresheet 1

	Poor		Fair		Good		Very Good		Excellent	
Professional appearance	1	2	3	4	5	6	7	8	9	10
Introduces self and shakes hands	1	2	3	4	5	6	7	8	9	10
Nonverbal communication (eye contact, facial expressiveness, body language)	1	2	3	4	5	6	7	8	9	10
Communicates effectively (open-ended questions, avoids jargon)	1	2	3	4	5	6	7	8	9	10
Establishes rapport with patient (empathy, appears nonjudgmental)	1	2	3	4	5	6	7	8	9	10
Allows patient to speak without being interrupted	1	2	3	4	5	6	7	8	9	10
Listens and seems to understand patient's concerns	1	2	3	4	5	6	7	8	9	10
Overall professionalism	1	2	3	4	5	6	7	8	9	10

Total Score:

Passing score for CIS section is 56 points.

Spoken English Proficiency (SEP) Scoresheet

Please rate each of the following items on a scale from 1–10.
These items may be completed by either the standardized patient or another student.

Scoresheet 2

	Poor		Fair		Good		Very Good		Excellent	
Examiner is articulate and easily understood	1	2	3	4	5	6	7	8	9	10
Pronunciation (words pronounced correctly; accent does not hinder communication)	1	2	3	4	5	6	7	8	9	10
Word choice is appropriate	1	2	3	4	5	6	7	8	9	10
Ability to communicate without excessive listener effort required to understand questions or responses	1	2	3	4	5	6	7	8	9	10
Patient's ability to understand the examiner	1	2	3	4	5	6	7	8	9	10
Examiner's ability to understand the patient	1	2	3	4	5	6	7	8	9	10

Total Score:

Passing score for SEP section is 42 points.

Acute Visual Change

History

In any patient complaining of visual change, the chronicity of the visual change should be determined. For the purposes of this chapter, we will focus on the patient with acute visual change. The differential diagnosis is guided primarily by the history to be obtained, which can then be supported by the physical examination. Key elements of this history include the following:

- Baseline visual status, which is most useful if there is a prior documented visual status. If not, the patient can be questioned about this, though patients may have gradual visual loss that may not be noticed until a certain threshold is reached.
- Monocular or binocular vision loss
- Transient or persistent vision loss
- Timeline. It should be determined whether the visual loss was abrupt or whether it occurred over hours, days, or weeks.
- Presence of floaters. Floaters may be described by the patient as fine dots, veils, cobwebs, clouds, or strings.
- History of trauma to the eye
- Eye pain
- Redness of the eye
- Past medical history
- Family history of visual problems
- Review of systems including headache, photophobia, vertigo

Physical Examination

Key aspects of the physical examination are outlined in the following list. If there are any aspects of the examination that are not clearly understood, we recommend that you consult a basic ophthalmology textbook for further details.

- **Distance visual acuity** testing using a Snellen eye chart.
- **External inspection of the lids, palpebral fissures, and the surrounding tissues.** The conjunctiva and sclera should be inspected using a penlight or the light from the ophthalmoscope. The conjunctiva and sclera should be examined by asking the patient to look up while the lower lid is retracted and to look down while the upper lid is raised.
- **Pupillary reaction testing** examines the patient's direct and consensual papillary reactions to light. The direct pupillary reaction is tested by directing the penlight at one eye to determine if the pupil constricts normally. The test is then repeated for the unaffected eye. To test the consensual pupillary reaction to light, the penlight is directed at one eye, and the other pupil is watched to see if it also constricts, indicating a normal consensual response. The test is then repeated on the other eye.
- **Ocular motility testing** should be performed to determine that ocular motility is intact in the six cardinal fields of gaze:
    - Right
    - Left
    - Right and up
    - Right and down
    - Left and up
    - Left and down
- **Ophthalmoscopy** involves several important steps:
    - The red reflex should be visualized. The eye is examined at a distance of 1 foot through the ophthalmoscope, and a red reflex should be produced by light reflecting off the fundus. The red reflex should be evenly colored and not interrupted by shadows.
    - The optic disk and cup as well as the retinal nerves and arteries should be viewed through the ophthalmoscope.
    - The retinal background color and the macula should be visualized. The retina should be a uniform red-orange color while the macula appears darker than the surrounding retina.
- **Intraocular pressure** using a Schiötz tonometer or a Tono-Pen should be determined when glaucoma is suspected. For the purposes of the Step 2 CS, intraocular pressure measurement should not be necessary.
- **Anterior chamber depth assessment** is measured because a shallow anterior chamber may indicate narrow-angle glaucoma. To determine anterior chamber depth, light is shone from the temporal side of the head across the front of the eye using a penlight. Then the nasal aspect of the iris is examined. If more than two-thirds of the nasal iris is in shadow, the chamber is probably shallow and the angle narrow, indicating the possibility of narrow-angle glaucoma.
- **Confrontation field testing** is used to measure visual status in each of the four quadrants of the

visual field. The examiner stands in front of the patient, and the patient is asked to cover the left eye while the examiner closes the right eye. The patient is asked to fixate on the examiner's left eye while counting the examiner's fingers in each of the four quadrants of vision. The examination is then repeated in the right eye.

- **Color vision testing** probably will not be required for the purposes of the Step 2 CS. However, it should be noted that color vision abnormalities, though usually inherited, may be acquired in patients with retinal or optic nerve disorders.
- **Upper lid eversion** allows an examination of the under side of the lid for the presence of a foreign body. The examiner gently grasps the eyelashes of the upper lid, and the patient is asked to look down. A cotton-tipped swab is used to press down gently over the upper lid while the eyelashes are pulled up. This action should evert the lid and allow the examiner to visualize the conjunctival aspect of the upper lid.
- **Fluorescein staining** of the cornea is used to diagnose defects of the corneal epithelium. Fluorescein is applied to the palpebral conjunctiva. The eye is then viewed under cobalt-blue light (Wood's lamp). Areas of bright-green staining mark denuded epithelium, indicating corneal abrasion or diseased epithelium.

Differential Diagnosis of Acute Visual Loss

The following list provides a differential diagnosis of acute visual loss. Though each of the following entities should be well understood, we have highlighted the diagnoses that we feel are most likely to appear on an examination such as the Step 2 CS. Following this list is a description and management plan for each of these processes.

1. Acute discovery of chronic visual loss
2. Central retinal vein occlusion
3. Corneal edema
4. Cortical blindness
5. **Giant cell arteritis**
6. Hyphema
7. Ischemic optic neuropathy
8. Macular disease
9. Occipital lobe transient ischemic attack (TIA) or infarction (or TIA or infarction in the middle cerebral artery distribution)
10. Ocular migraine
11. Optic neuritis
12. Rapidly developing cataract
13. **Retinal artery occlusion** (may result in TIA or infarction)
14. **Retinal detachment**
15. Trauma
16. Vitreous hemorrhage

Specific Causes of Acute Visual Loss

Acute Discovery of Chronic Visual Loss

Presentation: Some patients may have chronic progressive visual loss that presents as acute visual loss. If vision in one eye is normal, the eyes can function together, producing negligible visual disturbance until a certain threshold of visual loss is reached in the affected eye.

Examination: Obtaining previous records of eye examinations may aid in reaching this diagnosis.

Treatment: Ophthalmology consultation should be obtained.

Central Retinal Vein Occlusion

Presentation: Central retinal vein occlusion typically presents with severe visual loss usually in an older patient with hypertension and arteriosclerotic vascular disease.

Examination: Fundus examination is unique and reveals dilated and tortuous veins, flame-shaped hemorrhages, and cotton-wool spots.

Treatment: The prognosis for vision is poor. There is no real acute management, and this condition is not an ophthalmic emergency. Follow-up by an ophthalmologist should be arranged, because retinal laser photocoagulation may be used to prevent neovascular glaucoma.

Corneal Edema

Presentation: Corneal edema may be caused by any disease process that damages the corneal endothelium. Causes of corneal edema include acute glaucoma, herpes infection, and hypoxia due to contact lens use.

Examination: Examination with a slit-lamp may reveal clouding in the cornea.

Treatment: Therapy is directed at the underlying cause of the edema. Topical steroids may be used, but consultation with an ophthalmologist is recommended in cases of corneal edema.

Cortical Blindness

Presentation: Cortical blindness is an abnormality in vision caused by bilateral impairment of the occipital cortex vision centers. The papillary reaction to light remains intact, but vision is lost, and the patient may not be aware of the loss of vision. Transient cortical blindness has been observed in children following head trauma. In adults with cortical blindness, the condition either improves or is a sign of severe neurologic damage.

Examination: Loss of vision bilaterally on vision testing until intact pupillary responses to light.

Treatment: Neurology consultation is recommended.

Giant Cell Arteritis (Temporal Arteritis)

Presentation: Giant cell arteritis typically presents in a patient over the age of 60 with complaints of malaise, headache, scalp tenderness, pain in the jaw with chewing, and limb girdle pain. Jaw claudication is a classic and highly specific symptom. Vision loss may be present or impending.

Examination: Examination may reveal tenderness over the temporal arteries. An erythrocyte sedimentation rate (ESR) should be obtained immediately in the patient suspected of having giant cell arteritis. The ESR typically is elevated, often in excess of 60 mm per hour.

Treatment: Consists of high-dose systemic corticosteroids and immediate referral to an ophthalmologist for further management.

Hyphema

Presentation: Hyphema is blood in the anterior chamber, and any significant hyphema can reduce vision. Hyphema usually results from trauma to the eye, but may occur while the patient sleeps, perhaps as the result of subconsciously rubbing the eye.

Examination: Examination reveals blood in the anterior chamber of the eye.

Treatment: Small hyphemas are treated conservatively with monitoring for resolution. A hyphema filling more than 5% of the anterior chamber usually is treated with bed rest and steroid drops for 5 days. If steroid drops are to be used, ophthalmologic consultation is suggested.

Ischemic Optic Neuropathy

Presentation: Ischemic optic neuropathy occurs as the result of interruption of blood flow in the short posterior ciliary arteries that supply the optic disk. This condition results in a severe loss of vision that occurs suddenly or over several days. The vision loss is predominantly in the superior or inferior visual fields, a pattern termed *altitudinal.*

Examination: Examination reveals a pale, swollen optic disk, often accompanied by splinter hemorrhages and an afferent papillary defect.

Treatment: Patients suspected of having ischemic optic neuropathy should be referred for ophthalmologic evaluation.

Macular Disease

Presentation: Macular degeneration is the most common cause of legal blindness in persons older than 60 years in the United States. Macular degeneration typically is a slow, chronic process. However, in the "wet" form of the disease (which makes up less than 10% of macular degeneration), subretinal neovascularization occurs, which can result in bleeding and sudden visual loss. The patient may complain of vision loss with metamorphopsia, in which straight lines appear to bend.

Examination: Examination may reveal a dark green area or bright red blood in the retina.

Treatment: Patients suspected of having subretinal bleeding secondary to macular disease should receive prompt ophthalmologic evaluation.

Occipital Lobe TIA or Infarction (or Infarction in the Middle Cerebral Artery Distribution)

Presentation: Occlusion of one of the posterior cerebral arteries may result in occipital lobe infarction, which produces a homonymous hemianopia, a loss of vision on one side of both visual fields. Infarction in the distribution of the middle cerebral artery may also produce vision loss manifested as a hemianopia. However, because the middle cerebral artery supplies the motor cortex, other neurologic signs are usually present.

Examination: Examination may reveal a visual field defect.

Treatment: Patients with suspected infarction should be treated as having a cerebrovascular accident, which is covered in Chapter 18.

Ocular Migraine

Presentation: Retinal migraines are a distinct entity within the International Headache Society's diagnostic scheme and are also termed "ocular migraine," "ophthalmic migraine," and "headache with monocular blindness." They are defined as the occurrence of at least two attacks of monocular scotoma or blindness lasting less than 1 hour and associated with headache within 1 hour of the event, occurring in the absence of ocular or structural vascular disorder. The pathophysiology is thought to be retinal or ophthalmic nerve hypoperfusion.

Examination: Examination may reveal transient visual loss in one eye.

Treatment: Ocular migraines are treated as migraine headaches.

Optic Neuritis

Presentation: Optic neuritis typically affects younger patients and may present as monocular loss of vision over hours to days. The vision loss often is accompanied with pain during movements of the eye.

Examination: The general eye exam reveals poor vision in the affected eye, and an afferent papillary defect may be present. Ophthalmoscopy is unremarkable.

Treatment: A patient suspected of having optic neuritis should be seen by an ophthalmologist.

Rapidly Developing Cataract

Presentation: Though most cataracts develop slowly, certain conditions may result in rapid progression of a cataract and result in vision loss. Sudden changes in serum electrolytes or glucose may alter hydration of the lens, causing fluctuations in refractive error, which produces visual changes.

Examination: Examination reveals a hazy lens and decreased visibility of the fundus by ophthalmology.

Treatment: Treatment is directed at the underlying metabolic derangement.

Retinal Artery Occlusion

Presentation: Retinal vascular occlusion results in a transient or permanent sudden loss of vision. Amaurosis fugax, a transient monocular visual loss due to arterial insufficiency, often is due to an embolus, and should lead to investigation of the ipsilateral carotid circulation. Central retinal artery occlusion presents as a sudden, painless, and often complete visual loss.

Examination: Examination may reveal the characteristic "cherry-red spot," in which the normal fovea stands in significant contrast to a pale retina. Central retinal artery occlusion is a true ophthalmic emergency and warrants immediate treatment by an ophthalmologist.

Branch retinal artery occlusion presents as partial vision loss, as only a branch of the central retinal artery is occluded. An embolus, likely from the ipsilateral carotid artery, is the most common cause of branch retinal artery occlusion. When this occurs, the carotid artery should be imaged.

Treatment: Suspected branch retinal artery occlusion also requires immediate ophthalmologic consultation.

Retinal Detachment

Presentation: The patient with retinal detachment typically complains of flashing lights in the affected eye followed by large numbers of floaters and a shade over the vision in the affected eye. The patient with retinal detachment may have a history of posterior vitreous detachment, a benign condition resulting in floaters. The incidence of retinal detachment increases with advancing age.

Examination: If retinal detachment is suspected, the pupil should be dilated to facilitate the ophthalmoscopic examination. Ophthalmoscopy may reveal a retina that appears elevated or with folds in the normally smooth contour. However, ophthalmoscopy may be completely normal.

Treatment: If retinal detachment is suspected, prompt ophthalmologic consultation should be obtained.

Trauma

Presentation: Trauma may result in acute visual loss through multiple mechanisms. Hyphema, globe rupture, damage to the optic nerve, and intracranial processes may result in vision loss.

Examination: Findings on examination relate to the mechanism of injury. If globe rupture or damage to the optic nerve is suspected as the cause of vision loss, immediate consultation should be obtained from an ophthalmologist.

Treatment: If an intracranial process is suspected, appropriate imaging and neurologic or neurosurgical consultation should be obtained.

Vitreous Hemorrhage

Presentation: Vitreous hemorrhage may occur as the result of trauma or in any condition associated with retinal neovascularization, such as diabetes. Vitreous hemorrhage may also occur with subarachnoid hemorrhage. Vitreous hemorrhage may reduce vision either directly by placing opaque blood between the lens and the retina, or indirectly by causing retinal detachment.

Vitreous hemorrhage may be difficult to appreciate on exam, but if the lens appears clear and the red reflex cannot be seen, vitreous hemorrhage should be suspected.

Examination: Examination with a slit-lamp through a dilated pupil should be performed by an ophthalmologist.

Treatment: Suspected vitreous hemorrhage requires prompt ophthalmologic consultation.

REFERENCES

Asbury T, Sanitato JJ. In: Vaughan D, Asbury T, Riordan-Eva P, eds. General Ophthalmology, 15th ed. Stamford, CT, Appleton & Lange, 1999, p 351.

Berson FG. Basic Ophthalmology for Medical Students and Primary Care Residents, 6th ed. San Francisco: American Academy of Ophthalmology, 1993, pp 1–38.

Flood MT, Balazs EA. Hyaluronic acid content in the developing and aging human liquid and gel vitreous. Invest Ophthalmol Vis Sci 1977;16(suppl):67.

Foos RY, Wheeler NC. Vitreoretinal juncture. Synchysis senilis and posterior vitreous detachment. Ophthalmology 1982;89:1502–1512.

Gariano RF, Kim CH. Evaluation and management of suspected retinal detachment. Am Fam Phys 2004;69;1691–1698.

Headache and Classification Committee of the International Headache Society. Classification and diagnostic criteria for headache disorders, cranial neuralgias, and facial pain. Cephalgia 1988; 8(suppl 7):1–96.

Hikichi T, Trempe CL. Relationship between floaters, light flashes, or both, and complications of posterior vitreous detachment. Am J Ophthalmol 1994; 117:593–598.

Lewinshtein D, Shevell MI, Rothner AD. Familial retinal migraines. Pediatr Neurol 2004;30:356–357.

Liesegang TJ. In: Bartley GB, Liesegang TJ, eds. Essentials of Ophthalmology. Philadelphia, Lippincott, 1992, pp 70–71.

Newell FW. In: Ophthalmology Principles and Concepts. St. Louis, Mosby, 1996, pp 144, 320–321, 361–362.

Quillen DA. Common causes of vision loss in elderly patients. Am Fam Physician 1999;60:99–108.

Riordan-Eva P. In: Vaughan D, Asbury T, Riordan-Eva P, eds. General Ophthalmology, 15th ed. Stamford, CT, Appleton & Lange, 1999, p 256.

Rosenblatt BJ, Benson WE. In: Yanoff M, Duker JS, eds. Ophthalmology, 2nd ed. St. Louis, Mosby, 2004, pp 879–881.

Saadati HG, Sadun AA. In: Yanoff M, Duker JS, eds. Ophthalmology, 2nd ed. St. Louis, Mosby, 2004, pp 1384–1385.

Sanders MD, Graham EM. In: Vaughan D, Asbury T, Riordan-Eva P, eds. General Ophthalmology, 15th ed. Stamford, CT, Appleton & Lange, 1999, pp 290–292.

White PF, Scott CA. In: Yanoff M, Duker JS, eds. Ophthalmology, 2nd ed. St. Louis, Mosby, 2004, p 83.

"I Have an Elephant on My Chest"

Examinee Prompt

You are seeing this 57-year-old patient in the emergency department for a chief complaint of "chest pain." Please complete the following tasks:

- Obtain a focused history relevant to this patient's complaint
- Perform an appropriate physical examination

You will have 15 minutes to complete your visit with the patient. When you have all of the information that you need, you may leave the examination room. You do not need to explain your findings or your plan to the patient. Following your visit with the patient, please complete the following tasks:

- Write a "SOAP" (Subjective, Objective, Assessment and Plan)note, which should include your diagnosis. You will be provided with an electrocardiogram, and your findings/interpretation should be noted on the progress note.
- Outline your initial plan for the workup of this patient.

Vital Signs

Temperature .... 98.7° F

Blood pressure 152/92

Pulse 98

Respiratory rate 20

Patient Prompt

Background: You are a 57-year-old patient with 1 hour of substernal chest pain that began while mowing the lawn. You were driven to the emergency department by your spouse.

Chief Complaint: Chest pain

History of the Present Illness: 57-year-old patient with 1 hour of substernal squeezing chest pain. The chest pain began while mowing the lawn. No previous history of chest pain or cardiac problems. Some dyspnea and nausea. No vomiting, lightheadedness, or diaphoresis. No radiation of the pain.

Past Medical History: None

Past Surgical History: None

Gynecologic History: None or noncontributory

Medications: None

Allergies: No known drug allergies

Family History:
- Father with a history of prostate cancer, now status postprostatectomy
- Mother with hypertension
- Older brother with a cerebrovascular accident at age 64

Social History:
- Full-time work as a salesperson
- Married with three children
- Smokes 1/2 pack of cigarettes per day for 40 years
- Few beers on the weekends
- No illicit drug use

Review of Systems: Negative except as noted in the history of the present illness.

Additional Information: You are a relatively calm type of person but are moderately concerned about this chest pain. You noticed the pain while mowing the lawn but didn't initially think too much about it. When you mentioned it to your spouse, your spouse decided to bring you to the emergency department immediately.

There are no specific findings on the examination. Your overall demeanor is unremarkable, though you do have a chest pain intensity of 5 out of 10. As you are examined, it is not necessary to report any findings to the examiner.

Chest Pain Scoresheet

Subjective

- ❑ Onset of pain
- ❑ Nature of pain
- ❑ Radiation of pain
- ❑ Alleviating or exacerbating factors (such as activity/exercise)
- ❑ Associated cardiac symptoms (must ask at least three of the following: lightheadedness, nausea, vomiting, diaphoresis, palpitations, dyspnea)
- ❑ Past medical history
- ❑ Family medical history
- ❑ Smoking history

Objective

- ❑ General assessment
- ❑ Cardiovascular exam
- ❑ Evaluation of the neck veins and carotid arteries
- ❑ Pulmonary exam
- ❑ Abdominal exam
- ❑ Palpation of the chest wall
- ❑ Examination of the extremities

Assessment

- ❑ Acute coronary syndrome or acute myocardial infarction (must be included as one of the diagnoses)
- ❑ Credit for up to four of the items listed in the differential diagnosis of chest pain, provided in the text:
- ❑ Diagnosis #1
- ❑ Diagnosis #2
- ❑ Diagnosis #3
- ❑ Diagnosis #4

Plan (credit for up to five of the following)

- ❑ Electrocardiogram
- ❑ Serum cardiac marker levels
- ❑ Serum electrolytes
- ❑ Serum coagulation studies
- ❑ Pulse oximetry
- ❑ Chest x-ray
- ❑ IV access

Total Score: ____ / 25

Passing score for this station is 17 correct items.

Communication and Interpersonal Skills (CIS) Scoresheet

Please rate each of the following items on a scale from 1–10.
These items may be completed by either the standardized patient or another student.

Scoresheet 1

	Poor		Fair		Good		Very Good		Excellent	
Professional appearance	1	2	3	4	5	6	7	8	9	10
Introduces self and shakes hands	1	2	3	4	5	6	7	8	9	10
Nonverbal communication (eye contact, facial expressiveness, body language)	1	2	3	4	5	6	7	8	9	10
Communicates effectively (open-ended questions, avoids jargon)	1	2	3	4	5	6	7	8	9	10
Establishes rapport with patient (empathy, appears nonjudgmental)	1	2	3	4	5	6	7	8	9	10
Allows patient to speak without being interrupted	1	2	3	4	5	6	7	8	9	10
Listens and seems to understand patient's concerns	1	2	3	4	5	6	7	8	9	10
Overall professionalism	1	2	3	4	5	6	7	8	9	10

Total Score:

Passing score for CIS section is 56 points.

Spoken English Proficiency (SEP) Scoresheet

Please rate each of the following items on a scale from 1–10.
These items may be completed by either the standardized patient or another student.

Scoresheet 2

	Poor		Fair		Good		Very Good		Excellent	
Examiner is articulate and easily understood	1	2	3	4	5	6	7	8	9	10
Pronunciation (words pronounced correctly; accent does not hinder communication)	1	2	3	4	5	6	7	8	9	10
Word choice is appropriate	1	2	3	4	5	6	7	8	9	10
Ability to communicate without excessive listener effort required to understand questions or responses	1	2	3	4	5	6	7	8	9	10
Patient's ability to understand the examiner	1	2	3	4	5	6	7	8	9	10
Examiner's ability to understand the patient	1	2	3	4	5	6	7	8	9	10

Total Score:

Passing score for SEP section is 42 points.

Approach to the Patient With Chest Pain

Introduction

Evaluating a patient with chest pain is a challenge that the physician frequently encounters in various settings, including the office, the emergency department, and the hospital. The differential diagnosis of chest pain is broad and ranges from benign to potentially life-threatening. Obtaining a timely, thorough history is important because the lack of an immediately available definitive test poses diagnostic challenges. This chapter provides an approach to the evaluation of chest pain that will assist in differentiating the patient with cardiac chest pain from the patient with chest pain of another cause. The differential diagnosis of chest pain is reviewed, and the management of the patient with suspected cardiac chest pain is discussed.

Obtaining the History

In evaluating the patient with chest pain, it is vital to understand the typical presentations of typical cardiac chest pain as well as atypical chest pain. Typical chest pain related to an ischemic or anginal process usually presents as pressure, crushing, tightness, aching, or a viselike sensation. The patient may describe the proverbial "elephant sitting on my chest." The pain typically has a total duration between 5 and 15 minutes, and the pain usually takes several minutes to reach maximal intensity before it begins to improve. The pain may radiate to the arm, the jaw, or the back. The chest pain may also be accompanied by associated symptoms such as nausea, vomiting, dyspnea, lightheadedness, and diaphoresis. The patient may also complain of distress, anxiety, or a sense of impending doom. Typically, the pain increases with exertion and improves with rest or nitroglycerin.

Atypical chest pain is a term that refers to chest pain not believed to originate from cardiac origin. Symptoms essentially are those that do not fall into the category of typical angina. For example, pain that occurs suddenly and that lasts for only a few minutes, pain that resolves with activity, pleuritic chest pain, and pain that occurs with movement of the chest wall may all be classified as atypical chest pain. Additionally, indigestion-type pain is a common cause of atypical chest pain that should be considered, especially with complaints of heartburn or midepigastric discomfort.

An important point to remember is that although the symptoms just mentioned are classified as atypical chest pain, they may also be associated with cardiac ischemia. Sharp or stabbing pain, the sensation of indigestion, and pain radiating only to the right arm have been found in patients with documented myocardial infarction. The elderly population provides an additional diagnostic challenge because so-called atypical symptoms become more common manifestations of cardiac ischemia in older individuals. In addition to chest pain and dyspnea, chest pain in the elderly may present as syncope, altered mental status, weakness, giddiness, and cerebrovascular accidents. Patients with diabetes and coronary disease may present with similar atypical symptoms or may have silent ischemia. As such, these symptoms should be used to guide the assessment of the patient with chest pain, but should not ultimately define the assessment.

Risk Factors for Coronary Artery Disease

Risk factors predisposing to the development of coronary artery disease (CAD) must be considered in the patient presenting with chest pain. The classic risk factors for CAD include advancing age, male gender, cigarette smoking, diabetes, hyperlipidemia, hypertension, and a family history of premature CAD. Sedentary lifestyle, obesity, and type A personality traits also are associated with the development of CAD. In addition to these traditional coronary risk factors, a variety of other hereditary and acquired medical conditions may contribute to the development of CAD. Some of these conditions include the following:

- Elevated homocysteine levels
- Human immunodeficiency virus (HIV) infection
- End-stage renal disease
- Rheumatoid arthritis
- Systemic lupus erythematosis
- Thrombophilias such as factor V Leyden
- Elevated C-reactive protein levels
- Cocaine use (which can produce myocardial infarction in the absence of atherosclerotic disease through vasoconstriction alone)

Physical Examination

The physical examination in the patient with chest pain should include the following components:

- General assessment of the patient. The patient with cardiac ischemia may appear restless, diaphoretic, anxious, or tachypneic.

- Cardiovascular examination. A thorough cardiovascular examination should be performed on all patients complaining of chest pain. Acute ischemia may present with a new murmur, an increased first heart sound, a third heart sound, a fourth heart sound, or a pericardial friction rub. A large area of ischemia or infarction may result in findings of congestive heart failure, which include jugular venous distention or hepatomegaly. Finally, a large infarction may result in cardiogenic shock.
- Pulmonary examination. The pulmonary exam may be significant for crackles or wheezing in the patient presenting with congestive heart failure due to ischemia or infarction. Asymmetric breath sounds may indicate pneumothorax.
- Examination of the chest wall. The chest wall should be palpated for any evidence of musculoskeletal tenderness or other causes of chest wall pain such as malignancy or metastatic disease.
- Examination of the back. As with the examination of the chest wall, examination of the back may reveal musculoskeletal causes of the patient's chest pain.
- Abdominal examination. The abdomen should be carefully examined as any intra-abdominal process may present with pain that is referred to the chest, particularly in the older patient.

Differential Diagnosis of Chest Pain

The differential diagnosis of chest pain can be daunting. However, most cases of chest pain actually represent a much smaller list of disease processes. The differential diagnosis does not need to be memorized, but the clinician should be familiar with each of the potential causes so as to consider them in the workup of the patient with chest pain. For the purposes of focusing on the evaluation of the patient with chest pain, we present a list of the more common causes of chest pain:

Cardiovascular Causes

- Acute ischemic coronary syndrome (angina, myocardial infarction)
- Pericarditis
- Aortic dissection

Gastroenterologic Causes

- Gastroesophageal reflux (GERD), the most common cause of noncardiac chest pain
- Biliary colic
- Cholecystitis
- Esophageal dysmotility
- Hepatitis
- Pancreatitis
- Splenomegaly
- Pneumoperitoneum
- Superior vena cava syndrome

Pulmonary Causes

- Pulmonary embolism
- Pleurisy
- Pneumothorax
- Pneumonia
- Hyperventilation

Musculoskeletal Causes

- Costochondritis
- Cervical and thoracic spine disease
- Pectoral muscle syndromes
- Thoracic outlet syndrome

Soft Tissue Causes

- Herpes zoster
- Breast disorders

Psychiatric Causes

- Anxiety-panic disorder
- Depression
- Hypochondriasis
- Munchausen syndrome

Electrocardiographic Findings Suggestive of Cardiac Ischemia and Infarction

The electrocardiogram (ECG) is a useful tool employed in the initial evaluation of the patient with chest pain. The ECG may provide evidence of acute coronary ischemia and can also reveal clues to other clinical syndromes causing chest pain such as acute pericarditis and pulmonary embolus. The interpretation of the ECG is beyond the scope of this text. If you do not feel comfortable with your ability to adequately interpret the ECG, we recommend that you consult a textbook on this topic.

An important point to remember is that the ECG has several shortcomings that may limit its utility in the evaluation of chest pain. First, many cases of cardiac ischemia may present with a normal ECG or with nonspecific changes. These ECGs may remain normal or may evolve over time into electrocardiographic findings more typical of cardiac ischemia. Second, electrocardiographic abnormalities associated with cardiac ischemia may be masked by patterns such as left bundle branch block (LBBB), left ventricular hypertrophy, and ventricular paced rhythm.

There are several characteristic findings on the ECG that suggest cardiac ischemia. These include the following:

- The hyperacute T wave may appear as early as 30 minutes after the onset of coronary occlusion and usually evolves rapidly to become ST segment elevation.
- ST segment elevation represents a progressing infarction.
- ST segment depression represents myocardial ischemia, but may also occur with infarction. ST segment depression in the right precordial leads can represent infarction of the posterior wall of the myocardium.
- Reciprocal ST segment depression occurs in leads separate from leads reflecting ST segment elevation. This constellation of findings identifies a patient with acute myocardial infarction who is at increased risk of a poor outcome.
- T wave inversion may result from myocardial ischemia.
- Q waves usually represent previous myocardial infarction.

As previously mentioned, pericarditis and pulmonary embolus may also be suggested by certain findings on the ECG:

- Acute pericarditis may manifest as ST segment elevations, usually <5 mm in height, in numerous leads.
- Pulmonary embolism may be revealed on ECG with the classic changes of an S wave in lead I, a Q wave in lead III, and T wave inversion in lead III.

Managing the Patient with Suspected Cardiac Ischemia

The patient who has chest pain suggestive of cardiac ischemia should receive an immediate assessment consisting of the following measures:

- Measurement of vital signs
- Measurement of oxygen saturation
- IV access
- 12-lead ECG
- Focused history and physical exam
- Initial serum cardiac marker levels
- Electrolyte and coagulation studies
- Portable chest radiograph

Following the initial assessment, the following treatments should be administered to the patient. These may be remembered with the mnemonic **MONA**: Morphine, Oxygen, Nitroglycerin, Aspirin.

- Oxygen at 4 L per minute
- Aspirin 160 to 325 mg chewed
- Nitroglycerin sublingual or spray
- Morphine intravenously if pain is not relieved with nitroglycerin

The ECG should then be reviewed, and based upon the findings the patient can be placed into one of three treatment groups:

1. **ST elevation myocardial infarction (MI)**. The ECG in this group reveals ST segment elevations or new or presumably new LBBB which is strongly suspicious for MI. The following adjunctive treatments should be instituted:
    - β-blockers IV
    - Nitroglycerin IV
    - Heparin IV
    - HMG-CoA reductase inhibitors (statin medication)
    - Angiotensin-converting enzyme (ACE)-inhibitors after 6 hours or when stable

If the time from onset of symptoms is <12 hours, reperfusion should be attempted based on local resources. Options include angiography, angioplasty plus stent, or fibrinolytic therapy. It should be noted that there are contraindications to fibrinolytic therapy and that fibrinolytic therapy drops to a Class IIa intervention in patients over age 75.

If the time from onset of symptoms is >12 hours, the patient is no longer a candidate for reperfusion because studies indicate only a small benefit. If the patient is clinically stable, admission to a cardiac care unit or monitored bed should be obtained, and the patient treated with adjunctive treatments as indicated (β-blockers, nitroglycerin IV, heparin IV). However, if the patient has persistent symptoms or ST elevation, fibrinolytic therapy or angioplasty with stenting may provide some benefit.

2. **High-risk unstable angina or non-ST elevation MI**. The ECG in this group reveals ST depression or dynamic T wave inversion, both of which are strongly suspicious for ischemia. The following adjunctive treatments should be instituted:
    - Heparin (either unfractionated or low-molecular-weight heparin)
    - Aspirin 160 to 325 mg daily

- Glycoprotein IIb/IIIa receptor inhibitors
- Nitroglycerin IV
- β-blockers IV
- HMG-CoA reductase inhibitors (statin medication)

If the patient is clinically stable following these therapies, admission to a cardiac care unit or monitored bed should be obtained, and the patient treated with adjunctive treatments as indicated. However, if the patient has persistent symptoms or ST elevation, fibrinolytic therapy or angioplasty with stenting may provide some benefit.

3. **Intermediate or low-risk unstable angina**. The ECG in this group is nondiagnostic, revealing the absence of changes in the ST segments or T waves. If unstable angina or new-onset angina is suspected despite a nondiagnostic ECG, the patient should be treated as the patients in group number 2. Additionally, if the troponin is positive, the patient should be treated as the patients in group number 2.

All other patients with nondiagnostic ECGs should be monitored in a chest pain unit with serial ECGs and serial serum markers including troponin. Any evidence of ischemia or infarction warrants admission to a coronary care unit or monitored bed with adjunctive treatments started.

If there is no evidence of ischemia or infarction, the patient may be discharged with appropriate follow-up.

REFERENCES

Antman EM, Braunwald E. Acute myocardial infarction. In: Braunwald E: Heart Disease: A Textbook of Cardiovascular Medicine, 5th ed. Philadelphia, WB Saunders, 1997, p 1198.

Bayer A, Joginder S, Raafat F. Changing presentation of myocardial infarction with increasing old age. J Am Geriatr Soc 1986;266:2634–266.

Brady WJ Jr, Aufderheide TP, Chan T, Perron AD. Electrocardiographic diagnosis of acute myocardial infarction. Emerg Med Clin North Am 2001; 19:295–300.

Brody S, Slovis C, Wrenn K. Cocaine-related medical problems. Am J Med 1990;88:325–331.

Braunwald E. The history. In: Braunwald E, ed. Heart Disease: A Textbook of Cardiovascular Medicine, 5th ed. Philadelphia, WB Saunders, 1997, p 4.

Cummins RO, ed. Acute coronary syndromes: Patients with acute ischemic chest pain. In: ACLS Provider Manual. American Heart Association, Dallas, TX. 2001, pp 123–144.

Eslick GD, Fass R. Noncardiac chest pain: Evaluation and treatment. Gastroenterol Clin 2003;32:531–552.

Fruegard P, Launbjerg J, Hesse B, et al. The diagnosis of patients admitted with acute chest pain but without myocardial infarction: A population-based perspective. Am Heart J 1998;136:1028–1034.

Jones ID, Slovis CM. Diagnosis and treatment of acute myocardial infarction: Emergency department evaluation of the chest pain patients. Emerg Med Clin North Am 2001;19:269–282.

Kontos J, Jesse R. Evaluation of chest pain in the emergency department. Curr Prob Cardiol 1997;22(4): 149–236.

Lee T, Cook F, Weisberg M, et al. Acute chest pain in the emergency room identification and examination of low risk patients. Arch Intern Med 1985;145:65–69.

Nadelman J, Frishman W, Ooi W, et al. Prevalence, incidence and prognosis of recognized and unrecognized myocardial infarction in persons aged 75 years or older: The Bronx aging study. Am J Cardiol 1990;66:533–537.

Spin JM. Early use of statins in acute coronary syndromes. Curr Cardiol Rep 2002;4:289–297.

"I Passed Out"

Examinee Prompt

You are seeing this 67-year-old patient in the emergency department for a chief complaint of "passing out." Please complete the following tasks:

❑ Obtain a focused history relevant to this patient's complaint.

❑ Conduct an appropriate physical examination.

You have 15 minutes to complete your visit with the patient. When you have all of the information that you need you may leave the examination room. Following your visit with the patient, you will be asked to write a complete progress note, including a five-item differential diagnosis as well as a diagnostic plan. You will have 10 additional minutes to complete this portion of the progress note.

Vital Signs

Temperature .... 98.8°F
Blood pressure 134/78
Pulse 70
Respiratory rate 14

Patient Prompt

Background: You are a 67-year-old patient who had an unwitnessed episode of syncope as described below. You are moderately concerned about this episode as it has never occurred before.

Chief Complaint: "I passed out."

History of the Present Illness: 67-year-old patient with witnessed episode of syncope. The event occurred about 9 PM (less than 1 hour ago) as you arose from your desk where you had been working for the previous 2 hours. As you arose from the desk, you felt warm, lightheaded, and slightly nauseated. It seemed that your vision dimmed, and then you passed out. You awoke as your spouse came to your aid, and there was no confusion following this event. Your spouse witnessed the episode and did not note any seizure activity, tongue biting, or urinary incontinence. There was no head trauma. There was no associated headache, diplopia, or focal weakness. There were no associated cardiac symptoms such as chest pain, palpitations, or shortness of breath. You deny any previous history of syncope. You have not been dehydrated. You did eat a full dinner about 2 ½ hours prior to this episode, and you had two or three glasses of wine with dinner.

Past Medical History:
- Myocardial infarction age 58 with two vessel stenting
- Depression without any history of suicidal ideation

Past Surgical History: Cholecystectomy, appendectomy

Gynecologic History: Noncontributory

Medications:
- Atenolol 25 mg at bedtime
- Lisinopril 20 mg at bedtime
- Hydrochlorothiazide 25 mg every morning
- Aspirin 81 mg daily
- Paroxetine 20 mg daily

Allergies: No known drug allergies

Family History:
- Father died of Alzheimer's disease age 86
- Mother died of ovarian cancer age 77
- No siblings

Social History:
- Works full-time as a business consult
- Married with two grown daughters
- Drinks two to three glasses of wine per night with dinner
- No smoking
- No illicit drug use

Review of Systems: Negative except as previously mentioned

Additional Information: The cardiovascular examination for this patient is intended to be normal. The neurologic examination should be normal. You may state that each part of the examination is normal as the examiner performs each component of the exam.

Syncope Scoresheet

Subjective

- ❑ Situation in which syncope occurred (standing, upon rising, with micturition, etc.)
- ❑ Prodromal symptoms (nausea, lightheadedness, warmth, etc.)
- ❑ Associated cardiac symptoms (chest pain, palpitations)
- ❑ Associated neurologic symptoms (headache, diplopia)
- ❑ Presence of any witnessed seizure activity
- ❑ Postevent confusion or injury
- ❑ Previous history of syncope
- ❑ Past medical history
- ❑ Family history, particularly of syncope or sudden death
- ❑ Medications
- ❑ Alcohol use

Objective

- ❑ Vital signs noted on progress note
- ❑ Evidence of head trauma
- ❑ Auscultation of the heart
- ❑ Evaluation of the carotid arteries and jugular veins
- ❑ Assessment for confusion (orientation to person, place, time, etc.)
- ❑ Pupillary symmetry noted
- ❑ Evaluation for nystagmus
- ❑ Evaluation of gait
- ❑ Evaluation of balance

Assessment (one point for each reasonable item in the differential diagnosis, for a maximum of five points)

- ❑ Vasovagal syncope
- ❑ Carotid sinus hypersensitivity
- ❑ Cardiac arrhythmia
- ❑ Organic heart disease (valve disorder, cardiomyopathy, etc.)
- ❑ Medication effects
- ❑ Orthostatic hypotension
- ❑ Alcohol effects
- ❑ Transient ischemic attack
- ❑ Migraine headache
- ❑ Psychiatric disorder (pseudoseizure, panic disorder, major depression)
- ❑ Metabolic disorder (hypoglycemia, adrenal failure, etc.)
- ❑ Hypovolemia
- ❑ Hyperventilation

Plan (credit for up to five of the following)

- ❑ Obtain orthostatics
- ❑ Electrocardiogram (ECG)
- ❑ Admit for telemetry monitoring
- ❑ Labs (complete blood count [CBC], electrolytes, blood urea nitrogen [BUN], creatinine, glucose)
- ❑ Echocardiogram (due to prior history of myocardial infarction)
- ❑ Exercise treadmill test (due to prior history of myocardial infarction)
- ❑ Head computed tomography (CT) may be considered though is not necessary in this case
- ❑ Tilt table testing
- ❑ Carotid sinus massage
- ❑ Carotid artery ultrasonography is acceptable but not indicated in this case

Total score _____ / 30

Passing score for this station is 21 correct items.

Communication and Interpersonal Skills (CIS) Scoresheet

Please rate each of the following items on a scale from 1–10.
These items may be completed by either the standardized patient or another student.

Scoresheet 1

	Poor		Fair		Good		Very Good		Excellent	
Professional appearance	1	2	3	4	5	6	7	8	9	10
Introduces self and shakes hands	1	2	3	4	5	6	7	8	9	10
Nonverbal communication (eye contact, facial expressiveness, body language)	1	2	3	4	5	6	7	8	9	10
Communicates effectively (open-ended questions, avoids jargon)	1	2	3	4	5	6	7	8	9	10
Establishes rapport with patient (empathy, appears nonjudgmental)	1	2	3	4	5	6	7	8	9	10
Allows patient to speak without being interrupted	1	2	3	4	5	6	7	8	9	10
Listens and seems to understand patient's concerns	1	2	3	4	5	6	7	8	9	10
Overall professionalism	1	2	3	4	5	6	7	8	9	10

Total Score:

Passing score for CIS section is 56 points.

Spoken English Proficiency (SEP) Scoresheet

Please rate each of the following items on a scale from 1–10.
These items may be completed by either the standardized patient or another student.

Scoresheet 2

	Poor		Fair		Good		Very Good		Excellent	
Examiner is articulate and easily understood	1	2	3	4	5	6	7	8	9	10
Pronunciation (words pronounced correctly; accent does not hinder communication)	1	2	3	4	5	6	7	8	9	10
Word choice is appropriate	1	2	3	4	5	6	7	8	9	10
Ability to communicate without excessive listener effort required to understand questions or responses	1	2	3	4	5	6	7	8	9	10
Patient's ability to understand the examiner	1	2	3	4	5	6	7	8	9	10
Examiner's ability to understand the patient	1	2	3	4	5	6	7	8	9	10

Total Score:

Passing score for SEP section is 42 points.

Approach to the Patient with Syncope

Introduction

Syncope is a sudden, unexpected loss of consciousness associated with a loss of postural tone with spontaneous recovery. A syncopal event is one of the more dramatic and anxiety-provoking symptoms encountered by patients and often produces a diagnostic dilemma for the clinician. However, syncope is a common manifestation of numerous disorders with a final common pathway of insufficient cerebral blood flow to maintain consciousness. Syncope must be differentiated from other disorders of altered consciousness, including seizures, sleep disorders, metabolic disorders, vertigo, presyncope, and psychiatric disorders.

In the evaluation of syncope, proving a specific diagnosis is often difficult due to a lack of residual abnormalities on examination or on initial diagnostic studies. The clinician must remember that syncope is a symptom, and not a disease. By possessing an understanding of the common etiologies that cause syncope, the clinician can focus the history, physical examination, and diagnostic evaluation in each specific case. An understanding of the available diagnostic tests and their indications is imperative.

This chapter reviews the more common causes of syncope, as well as the important elements of a thorough, focused history and physical examination. A review of the available diagnostic modalities is provided, followed by a discussion of treatment options.

Differential Diagnosis

The differential diagnosis of syncope is broad, and prevalence varies depending upon research methods employed in each study. The most common causes of syncope are vasovagal syncope, arrhythmias, and orthostatic hypotension. One should remember that after a standard diagnostic evaluation, it has been determined that as many as 50% of patients have syncope of unknown cause.

The following is a selected differential diagnosis of syncope. The more common and important causes are in italics.

Reflex Mediated

1. *Vasovagal*
2. Situational (cough, defecation, micturition, swallow)
3. *Carotid sinus hypersensitivity*

Cardiac

1. *Arrhythmia*
2. Organic heart disease (valvular disease, hypertrophic cardiomyopathy, tamponade, etc.)

Orthostatic Hypotension (autonomic dysfunction)

1. Diabetes
2. Amyloidosis
3. Paraneoplastic neuropathies
4. Human immunodeficiency virus (HIV) infection
5. Guillain-Barré syndrome
6. Parkinson disease
7. Shy-Drager syndrome

Medication Effects

1. Anticholinergic agents
2. β-adrenergic blockers
3. α-agonists
4. Vasodilators
5. Antipsychotics
6. Antiparkinsonian agents
7. Narcotics

Neurologic Causes

1. Migraine headache
2. Transient ischemic attack

Metabolic Disorders

1. Adrenal failure
2. Hypoglycemia

Psychiatric Causes

1. Pseudoseizures
2. Syncope related to panic disorder, major depression, etc.

Other Causes

1. Hypovolemia
2. Hyperventilation
3. Seizure (not a true case of syncope)
4. Subclavian steal syndrome
5. *Unknown*

Obtaining the History

The history provides the core of the diagnostic evaluation in the patient with syncope and guides further evaluation. The following items are key elements of the history:

- Situation in which syncope occurred (upon standing, in a fearful situation, during micturition, with coughing, with exertion)
- Prodromal symptoms (lightheadedness, warmth, nausea, sweating)
- Associated cardiac symptoms (chest pain, palpitations, shortness of breath)
- Associated neurologic symptoms (focal neurologic symptoms, headache, diplopia)
- Witnessed events (tonic/clonic movements, tongue biting, urinary incontinence)
- Previous history of syncope
- Recent dehydration
- Postevent symptoms
  - Confusion may indicate seizure activity
  - Injuries related to a fall
  - Duration of recovery
- Past medical history, particularly:
  - History of cardiac disease, including coronary artery disease, arrhythmias, or cardiomyopathy
  - History of cerebrovascular ischemia
  - History of pulmonary embolism or pulmonary hypertension
  - History of gastrointestinal bleeding
- Family history of syncope or sudden death
- Medications
  - Especially antihypertensive agents, antidepressants, vasodilators, narcotic analgesics, Q-T prolonging agents (tricyclic antidepressants), and hypoglycemic agents
- Social history
  - Particularly alcohol or marijuana use
  - Smoking history that places the patient at risk for cardiopulmonary disease

Physical Examination

The physical examination in the setting of syncope should include the following components:

- Vital signs
- Evaluation for orthostatic hypotension (defined as at least a 20 mm Hg systolic or 10 mm Hg diastolic drop in blood pressure within 3 minutes of standing)
- Cardiovascular examination
  - Carotid bruits
  - Murmurs
  - Jugular venous distention
  - Loud S2
  - Presence of an S3
  - Pericardial friction rubs
  - Blood pressures in both the arms
- Neurologic evaluation
  - Mental status
  - Pupil symmetry
  - Evaluation for nystagmus
  - Gait
  - Balance

Diagnostic Testing

Basic Laboratory Testing: Basic laboratory testing such as CBC, electrolytes, BUN, creatinine, and glucose are indicated when an underlying disorder is suspected as the cause of syncope. When performed routinely, these tests have a low diagnostic yield. In women of childbearing age, pregnancy testing should be considered.

Electrocardiography: The ECG is used routinely in the evaluation of syncope, primarily to identify abnormalities that may suggest an underlying cardiac cause for the syncope. These important findings include evidence of conduction disorders (bundle branch block, first-degree heart block, and sinus bradycardia), signs of coronary artery disease, or left ventricular hypertrophy that may be associated with ventricular tachycardia.

Echocardiography: The utility of echocardiography lies in its ability to identify patients with underlying cardiac conditions that are risk factors for ventricular tachycardia, such as prior myocardial infarction or cardiomyopathy. Echocardiography does not need to be performed routinely. Rather, the role of echocardiography is to rule out a cardiac cause of syncope in patients with suspected cardiac disease, as well as to quantify the degree of cardiac disease when it exists. In patients with exertional syncope, echocardiography can help exclude hypertrophic cardiomyopathy and aortic stenosis.

Exercise Tolerance Testing: The utility of an exercise test lies with confirming and quantifying coronary artery disease in patients with syncope in whom coronary artery disease is suspected. In addition, exercise tolerance testing may be used to rule out coronary artery disease and exercise-induced arrhythmias in patients with exertional syncope.

Holter Monitoring: Holter monitoring or telemetry is recommended for patients with known or suspected cardiac disease or a suspected arrhythmic cause of syncope.

Transtelephonic Electrocardiogram Monitoring: A transtelephonic monitor is an ambulatory cardiac monitor that is activated by a patient at the onset of symptoms. Data is then transmitted by telephone to a central station for interpretation. These monitors are most useful in patients with frequent syncope and either no suspected cardiac disease or a negative cardiac evaluation. These monitors are particularly useful for elderly patients without structural heart disease who are considered at risk for bradyarrhythmias.

Insertable Loop Recorders: Insertable loop recorders, about the size of a pacemaker, are inserted into the chest wall and are activated by the patient at the onset of symptoms. The role of these recorders has not yet been fully defined. Insertable loop recorders may be useful in patients without evidence of neurocardiogenic syncope or organic heart disease and with infrequent episodes of syncope that make the use of an external loop recorder impractical.

Electrophysiology Studies: Electrophysiology (EP) studies are invasive tests that use electric stimulation to diagnose conduction disease or susceptibility for developing tachyarrhythmias. EP studies are most useful in the following situations:

- Patients with a suspected arrhythmic cause for their syncope and a history of known heart disease, especially previous myocardial infarction or congestive heart failure
- Patients with preexcitation syndromes such as Wolff-Parkinson-White syndrome
- Patients with a suspected bradyarrhythmic cause for syncope, particularly older patients

Electroencephalogram (EEG): The diagnostic yield of EEG is very low, and the EEG is indicated only when seizure is suspected, such as when there is a history of tonic-clonic movements, postevent confusion, or a known seizure history.

Computed Tomography: CT scanning of the head has a relatively low yield in patients with syncope. Head CT is not routinely indicated, but is recommended in patients with focal neurologic symptoms and signs. Additionally, it may be performed in patients with seizure activity and head trauma to rule out intracranial hemorrhage.

Tilt Table Testing: Tilt table testing can be useful in patients with recurrent unexplained syncope with a suspected neurocardiogenic cause, particularly when symptoms consistent with neurocardiogenic syncope are present (warmth, nausea, sweating, lightheadedness). Tilt table testing also may be useful in patients without cardiac disease or in whom cardiac testing has been negative.

Carotid Sinus Massage: Carotid sinus massage should be considered in selected patients 60 years or older with an otherwise nondiagnostic evaluation for syncope. In carotid sinus massage, gentle pressure is applied to the carotid sinus. A sinus arrest of 3 seconds or longer or a 50 mm Hg drop in systolic blood pressure during the maneuver indicates carotid sinus hypersensitivity.

Vascular Studies: Currently, there are no studies to assess the utility of carotid ultrasonography or transcranial Doppler in the evaluation of patients with syncope. Both tests add little in the evaluation of syncope. Carotid disease or vertebrobasilar disease significant enough to cause a loss of consciousness would be unlikely in the absence of other neurologic signs such as diplopia, dysarthria, or vertigo.

Psychiatric Evaluation: Psychiatric evaluation is recommended in patients with recurrent unexplained syncope if there is no cardiac disease or if the cardiac evaluation is negative. Young patients and patients with many prodromal symptoms are at higher risk of having an underlying psychiatric disorder associated with their episodes of syncope. One study of 72 patients found associated psychiatric disorders in 24% of these patients. The most commonly associated psychiatric disorders were panic disorder and major depression.

Approach to Diagnosis

Many algorithms exist for the evaluation of syncope, and most emphasize the importance of the history and physical examination in making an accurate diagnosis. A position paper published by the American College of Physicians presents the following important features in guiding diagnosis:

- Separate patients into diagnostic, suggestive, and unexplained categories on the basis of the history, physical examination, and ECG findings
- Separate patients with unexplained syncope further on the basis of age and the presence of organic heart disease or an abnormal ECG
- Use echocardiography and treadmill stress testing to evaluate and quantify the degree of heart disease
- Reserve Holter monitoring and electrophysiology studies for patients with confirmed heart disease
- Employ tilt testing, loop recorders, and psychiatric evaluation in patients with recurrent unexplained syncope and no suspected heart disease or a negative cardiac evaluation

Although algorithms may provide a guide for the evaluation of syncope, the various available algorithms each contain controversial elements. In addition, algorithms do not consider every clinical situation and are not designed to replace individual clinician judgment. It is our recommendation that the physician-in-training should understand the approach to the patient with syncope first, and then consult algorithms to focus the diagnostic evaluation.

Treatment Options

The treatment of syncope should be focused on the underlying etiology, such as cardiac arrhythmia, metabolic disorders, or migraine headache. The following discussion represents treatment options available for the treatment of neurocardiogenic syncope (vasovagal and situational syncope). Treatment should be proportional to the frequency and severity of syncope, with consideration given to the risk of physical injury and the amount of patient distress.

Education should be provided regarding the avoidance of triggering conditions such as warm environments, hot baths, dehydration, prolonged standing, large meals, rising after prolonged rest, and Valsalva maneuvers such as micturition. Additionally, the role of alcohol and certain medications in syncope should be emphasized. The patient also should be educated about the use of adequate salt and water intake to decrease syncopal episodes.

Four pharmacologic agents have been shown to be effective in reducing syncopal episodes in randomized clinical trials. These agents are atenolol, midodrine, paroxetine, and enalapril. Although not evaluated in clinical trials, the mineralocorticoid fludrocortisone has been used extensively in the treatment of syncope. Other agents that have been used but are not clinically proven include disopyramide, scopolamine, theophylline, and clonidine.

A pacemaker may provide some benefit in patients with predominantly cardioinhibitory forms of syncope, but it remains controversial as a widespread therapy. Pacemakers may be considered for patients with recurrent, medically refractory, neurally mediated syncope with a documented cardioinhibitory tilt table response.

Finally, in most states, it is the physician's duty to provide a confidential morbidity report to the department of motor vehicles regarding a patient's lapse in consciousness.

REFERENCES

Abboud FM. Neurocardiogenic syncope. N Engl J Med 1993;328:1117–1120.

Atkins D, Hanusa B, Sefcik T, et al. Syncope and orthostatic hypotension. Am J Med 1991;91:179–185.

Calkins H. Pharmacologic approaches to therapy for vasovagal syncope. Am J Cardiol 1999;84:20Q–25Q.

Cunningham R, Mikhail MG. Management of patients with syncope and cardiac arrhythmias in an emergency department observation unit. Emerg Med Clin North Am 2001;19:105–121.

Davis TL, Freemon FR. Electroencephalography should not be routine in the evaluation of syncope in adults. Arch Intern Med 1990;150:2027–2029.

Di Girolamo E, Di Iorio C, Sabatini P, et al. Effects of paroxetine hydrochloride, a selective serotonin reuptake inhibitor, on refractory vasovagal syncope: A randomized, double-blind, placebo-controlled study. J Am Coll Cardiol 1999;33:1227–1230.

Kaufmann H. Neurally mediated syncope: Pathogenesis, diagnosis, and treatment. Neurology 1995;45(suppl 5):S12–S18.

Kapoor WN. Syncope. N Engl J Med 2000;343: 1856–1862.

Linzer M, Yang EH, Estes 3rd NA, et al. Diagnosing syncope: Part 1: Value of history, physical examination and electrocardiography. Clinical efficacy assessment project of the American College of Physicians. Ann Intern Med 1997;126:989–996,

Linzer M, Yang EH, Estes 3rd NA, et al. Diagnosing syncope: Part 2. Unexplained syncope. Clinical efficacy project of the American College of Physicians. Ann Intern Med 1997;127:763–786.

Mahanonda N, Bhuripanyo K, Kangkagate C, et al. Randomized double-blind, placebo-controlled trial of oral atenolol in patients with unexplained syncope and positive upright tilt table test results. Am Heart J 1995;130:1250–1253.

Munro NC, McIntosh S, Lawson J, et al. Incidence of complications after carotid sinus massage in older patients with syncope. J Am Geriatr Soc 1994;42:1248–1251.

Schnipper JL, Kapoor WN. Diagnostic evaluation and management of patients with syncope. Med Clin North Am 2001;85:423–456.

Sutton R, Brignole M, Menozzi C, et al. Dual chamber pacing in the treatment of neurally mediated positive cardioinhibitory syncope: Pacemaker versus no therapy—a multicenter randomized study. The Vasovagal Syncope International Study (VASIS) investigators. Circulation 2000;102: 294–299.

Sutton R, Petersen M, Brignole M, et al. Proposed classification for tilt induced vasovagal syncope. Eur J Pacing Electrophysiol 1992;3:180–183.

Ward CR, Gray JC, Gilroy JJ, et al. Midodrine: A role in the management of neurocardiogenic syncope. Heart 1998;79:45–49.

Weimer LH. Syncope and orthostatic intolerance for the primary care physician. Primary Care Clin Office Pract 2004;31:175–199.

Zeng C, Zhu Z, Liu G, et al. Randomized, double-blind, placebo-controlled trial of oral enalapril in patients with neurally mediated syncope. Am Heart J 1998;136:852–858.

Zimetbaum P, Kim KY, Ho KK, et al. Utility of patient-activated cardiac event recorders in general clinical practice. Am J Cardiol 1997;79:371–372.

CASE 17

"Do I Have Appendicitis Again?"

Examinee Prompt

You are working in an outpatient clinic and are asked to see a patient with a complaint of abdominal pain. Please perform the following tasks:

- ❑ Obtain a focused history relevant to this patient's chief complaint.
- ❑ Perform an appropriate physical exam.
- ❑ Following the examination, write a complete progress note documenting your findings.
- ❑ Provide a differential diagnosis, noting your most likely diagnosis first.
- ❑ Document an initial diagnostic plan.

You have 15 minutes to complete your visit with the patient. You will have 10 additional minutes to complete the progress note.

Vital Signs

Temperature . . . . 98.6°F
Blood pressure 120/80
Heart rate 108
Respiratory rate 12

Patient Prompt

Background: You are a 28-year-old patient seeing this doctor today to evaluate your severe abdominal pain. The last time you experienced pain of this severity, you were diagnosed with appendicitis. Please be familiar with the case details below. You may offer any of the following information if specifically asked.

Chief Complaint: Right-sided abdominal pain

History of the Present Illness: 28-year-old man with sharp, severe, right-sided abdominal pain (10/10 in intensity) for the last 12 hours. The pain developed fairly abruptly on the right flank with some radiation to the groin. The urine is darker than usual, but there is no gross hematuria. A few minutes after the pain began it migrated to the right lower abdomen. Nausea was present but improved after two episodes of vomiting. The emesis consisted of food and water with no blood or bile. The pain comes in waves of severity ranging from a dull ache of 4/10 to a maximum of 10/10. There is no relation of the pain to meals or bowel movements, though neither has occurred since the pain began. You admittedly have not been drinking fluids to keep up with your rigorous exercise routine. The last bowel movement 2 days ago was normal. When the pain is at its worst you feel like you can't sit still. Hydrocodone-acetaminophen left over from a dental procedure has not reduced the pain at all. You are anxious to get the interview over with so that you can get some pain medication as soon as possible.

Past Medial History:
- Appendicitis age 14
- Otherwise healthy

Past Surgical History: Appendectomy at age 14

Medications:
- Hydrocodone-acetaminophen as above, no regular use. Took one dose 3 hours ago.
- Multivitamin daily
- Vitamin C 2500 mg orally daily. (You read somewhere it was good for you.)

Allergies: Penicillin, which causes a rash

Social History:
- Single
- Graduate student
- Sexually active, monogamous, heterosexual
- Three prior partners
- No tobacco, drugs, or alcohol

Family History: No history of kidney stones, renal failure, renal tubular acidosis, or gout

Review of Systems:
- No fevers, some chills associated with severe pain
- No upper respiratory tract infection symptoms

- No recent diarrhea
- No constipation
- No blood in stools and no black tarry stools
- No dysuria, frequency, urgency, hesitancy
- No prior trauma

Additional Information: Please act out the pertinent positives and negatives during the physical exam. A pelvic, genitourinary, and rectal exam will not be performed. The details of the physical exam are as follows:

- General appearance: moderately ill nontoxic, some distress from pain. Frequently shifts position due to discomfort.
- HEENT: unremarkable
- Neck: supple, no lymphadenopathy
- Cardiovascular: unremarkable except tachycardia at a rate of 105 to 115
- Pulmonary: unremarkable
- Abdomen: normal bowel sounds, flat, soft, moderate tenderness to palpation in the right lower quadrant, no rebound or guarding, nondistended. No pain with movement of the body or lower extremities.
- Back: right costovertebral angle tenderness

Abdominal Pain Scoresheet

Subjective

- ❑ Location of pain
- ❑ Onset (rapid vs. gradual)
- ❑ Severity, including use of pain scale
- ❑ Radiation
- ❑ Nature of pain (sharp, colicky, dull, etc.)
- ❑ Nausea/vomiting
- ❑ Anorexia
- ❑ Urinary symptoms (dysuria, hematuria)
- ❑ Diarrhea or constipation
- ❑ Melena or blood in stools
- ❑ Fever or chills
- ❑ Past medical/surgical history
- ❑ Medications
- ❑ Allergies to medications

Objective

- ❑ General appearance: should indicate some degree of patient discomfort
- ❑ Cardiovascular: note tachycardia
- ❑ Lungs: clear
- ❑ Abdomen (1 point for performing the abdominal exam, and up to 3 points total for the following items):
  - ❍ Soft, nontender, nondistended
  - ❍ Absence of rebound and guarding
  - ❍ Normal bowel sounds
  - ❍ Back: right costovertebral angle tenderness

Assessment (this diagnosis should be included)

- ❑ Urolithiasis

Plan

- ❑ Rectal exam
- ❑ Complete blood count (CBC)
- ❑ Blood urea nitrogen (BUN) and creatinine
- ❑ Urinalysis (UA)
- ❑ One of the following:
  - ❍ Computed tomography (CT) scan of abdomen and pelvis
  - ❍ Intravenous pyelography (IVP)
- ❑ The following are optional (no points added or subtracted):
  - ❍ Plain abdominal radiograph of *k*idney, *u*reters, *b*ladder (KUB)
  - ❍ Liver function tests
  - ❍ Abdominal ultrasound
- ❑ The following should not have been ordered (1 point deducted for each):
  - ❍ Surgical consultation
  - ❍ Magnetic resonance imaging (MRI)
  - ❍ Colonoscopy
  - ❍ Upper GI/barium swallow
  - ❍ Barium enema
  - ❍ *Helicobacter pylori* antibody
  - ❍ Hepatitis viral serology
  - ❍ Stool ova and parasites (O&P), white blood count (WBC), culture

Total Score ____ / 28

Passing score for this station is 19 correct items.

Communication and Interpersonal Skills (CIS) Scoresheet

Please rate each of the following items on a scale from 1–10.
These items may be completed by either the standardized patient or another student.

Scoresheet 1

	Poor		Fair		Good		Very Good		Excellent	
Professional appearance	1	2	3	4	5	6	7	8	9	10
Introduces self and shakes hands	1	2	3	4	5	6	7	8	9	10
Nonverbal communication (eye contact, facial expressiveness, body language)	1	2	3	4	5	6	7	8	9	10
Communicates effectively (open-ended questions, avoids jargon)	1	2	3	4	5	6	7	8	9	10
Establishes rapport with patient (empathy, appears nonjudgmental)	1	2	3	4	5	6	7	8	9	10
Allows patient to speak without being interrupted	1	2	3	4	5	6	7	8	9	10
Listens and seems to understand patient's concerns	1	2	3	4	5	6	7	8	9	10
Overall professionalism	1	2	3	4	5	6	7	8	9	10

Total Score:

Passing score for CIS section is 56 points.

Spoken English Proficiency (SEP) Scoresheet

Please rate each of the following items on a scale from 1–10.
These items may be completed by either the standardized patient or another student.

Scoresheet 2

	Poor		Fair		Good		Very Good		Excellent	
Examiner is articulate and easily understood	1	2	3	4	5	6	7	8	9	10
Pronunciation (words pronounced correctly; accent does not hinder communication)	1	2	3	4	5	6	7	8	9	10
Word choice is appropriate	1	2	3	4	5	6	7	8	9	10
Ability to communicate without excessive listener effort required to understand questions or responses	1	2	3	4	5	6	7	8	9	10
Patient's ability to understand the examiner	1	2	3	4	5	6	7	8	9	10
Examiner's ability to understand the patient	1	2	3	4	5	6	7	8	9	10

Total Score:

Passing score for SEP section is 42 points.

Discussion of Urolithiasis

This case is a fairly classic presentation for a kidney stone (urolithiasis). The only significant point of consideration is that this patient did not have gross hematuria. However, a urinalysis (UA) would likely reveal microscopic hematuria. This patient's kidney stone case may have been precipitated by his poor hydration and intake of large amounts of vitamin C. Though popularized in the early 1990s, high-dose vitamin C can precipitate kidney stones, as it is bioconverted to oxalate, which is an element of many kidney stones. Referral to a urologist in this case is not necessarily indicated as there is no indication of infection, the stone is likely to pass spontaneously, and the patient's symptoms of pain/nausea are not yet deemed to be intractable.

A common mistake in treating urolithiasis is the inadequate use of higher potency analgesics. Hydrocodone and most nonsteroidal anti-inflammatory drugs (NSAIDs) are often ineffective for more severe pain.

Once the diagnosis of urolithiasis is made, straining the urine and sending the stone for analysis is helpful in diagnosing the specific stone etiology. This can greatly help the clinician in avoiding precipitants, advising dietary modifications, or prescribing prophylaxis (such as hydrochlorothiazide, potassium citrate, or allopurinol). A person with more than one episode of kidney stones should be worked up for an underlying etiology and offered prophylaxis.

Clinical pearl: Consider working up a patient for a kidney stone if an atypical pathogen is found on UA (e.g., *Proteus* spp.), if there is unexplained recurrent urinary tract infection, or for any patient with unexplained microscopic or gross hematuria.

A Systematic Approach to Acute Abdominal Pain

Introduction

A complaint of abdominal pain may present a seemingly overwhelming situation. The broad differential and potential for serious disease can be intimidating unless you have a fundamentally strong understanding of abdominal pain and strategy for dealing with each case. The additional stress of encountering this topic during an exam underscores the importance of having a routine and systematic approach to this clinical scenario. It will soon become very obvious that simply memorizing the extensive differential diagnosis of abdominal pain is in itself inadequate and troublesome.

Key Historical Features

Abdominal Colic: Recognizing a pattern of pain as "colicky" may be instrumental in arriving at a correct diagnosis. Colicky pain tends to be "crampy" in nature and usually waxes and wanes over time. Pain may alternate between severe and stabbing in nature and then subside to a dull ache. Unless there is concurrent peritoneal irritation (see below) the pain may be poorly localized. Colic suggests distention of a hollow viscus as seen in biliary, ureteral, and bowel disease.

Associated Symptoms: The symptoms that accompany abdominal pain may provide important clues to the correct diagnosis. Your familiarity with the review of systems of the various organ systems may be instrumental in helping narrow the differential diagnosis. For example:

- Symptoms made better or worse with meals or with bowel movements suggest a gastrointestinal or biliary tract etiology. Diarrhea, constipation, bright red blood per rectum, or melena also suggests the gastrointestinal tract as the source of pathology.
- Urinary symptoms such as dysuria, hematuria, frequency, hesitancy, urgency, or nocturia suggest genitourinary pathology.
- Vaginal bleeding or missed menses suggests gynecologic pathology.
- Constitutional symptoms such as fever, anorexia, and nausea and vomiting are much less specific. Their presence or absence does not suggest or rule out any particular disease state.

Radiation of Pain: In specific cases, abdominal pain may radiate to other areas, giving you possible clues to its etiology. For example:

- Pain radiating to the shoulders suggests a subdiaphragmatic process (e.g., hepatitis, splenic abscess, biliary disease).
- Pain radiating to the back may suggest a pancreatic, gastric, aortic, or renal etiology. The ascending and descending colon, which are retroperitoneal structures, may cause pain that radiates to the back or flank.
- Pain radiating to the groin or testes may suggest a perirenal process such as a kidney stone or perinephric abscess.

Formulate the Differential Diagnosis Based Upon Cross-Sectional Anatomy

Experienced clinicians often visualize the area of concern and the organ systems in the nearby vicinity. Consider the various diseases of those organs to formulate a differential diagnosis.

For example, right lower quadrant pain may involve the appendix, ovary (cyst), fallopian tube (tubo-ovarian abscess, ectopic pregnancy), colon (diverticulitis), ureter (stone), psoas muscle (abscess), abdominal wall (muscle strain, hernia), or testicle (epididymitis, torsion, orchitis). See Figure 1 for a differential diagnosis of abdominal pain based upon the quadrant involved.

Recognize Peritoneal Signs—"The Acute Abdomen"

An integral part of the evaluation of acute abdominal pain is the diagnosis of "the acute abdomen." When an acute abdomen is suspected, surgical evaluation often is necessary.

- Peritoneal signs are those physical exam findings that result from irritation or inflammation of the parietal peritoneum. The patient is

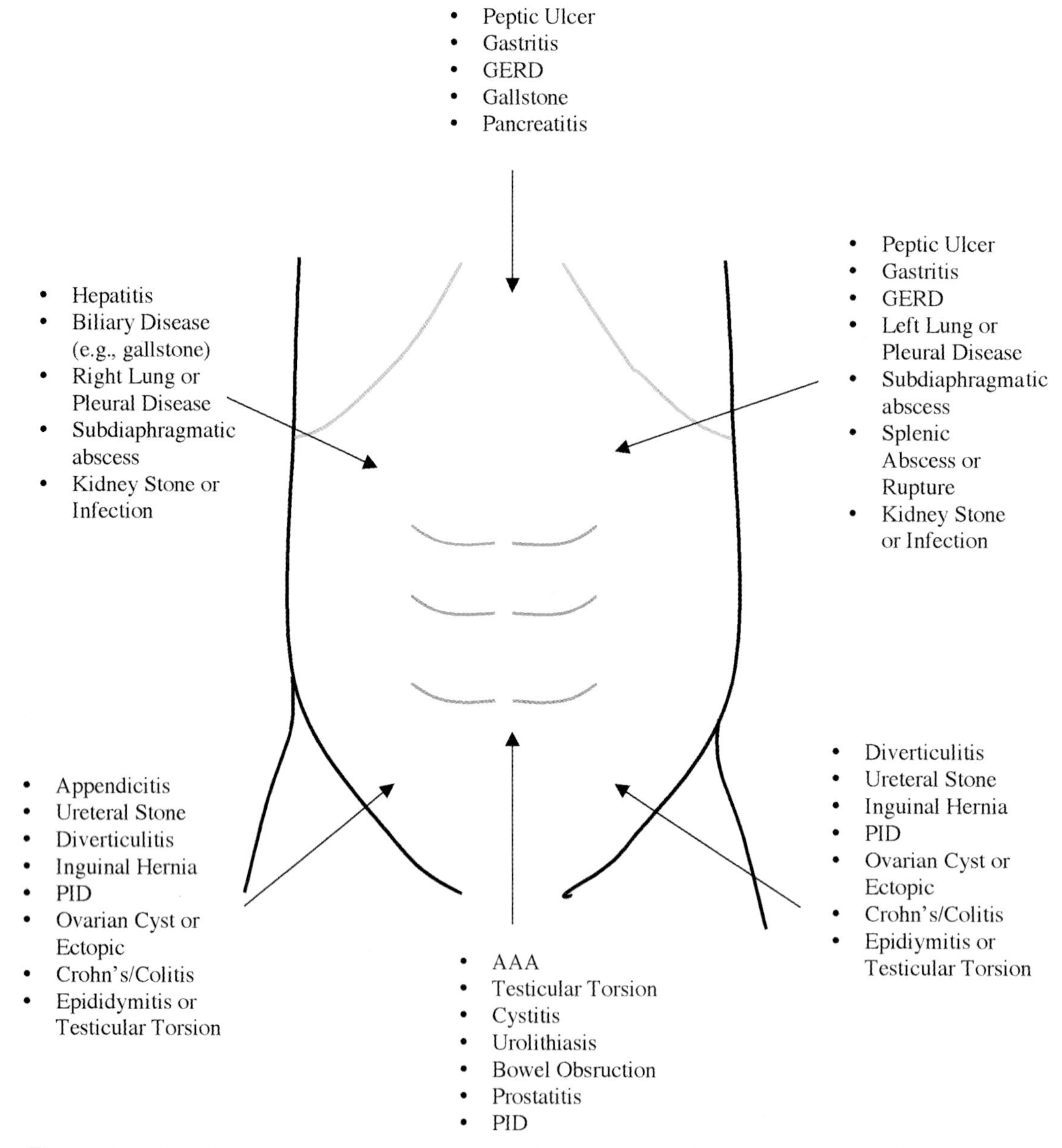

Figure 1. Differential diagnosis of abdominal pain by cross-sectional anatomy. AAA, abdominal aortic aneurysm; GERD, gatroesophageal reflux disease; PID, pelvic inflammatory disease.

often lying very still as any movement exacerbates the pain. Pain is often very well localized and reproducible with palpation. Guarding or rigidity (involuntary tensing of abdominal muscles), rebound tenderness (pain elicited with the release of deeper palpation), and referred tenderness (percussion or palpation of another area reproduces pain at the site of pathology) are usually present. Other methods of reproducing peritoneal pain include extension at the hip (psoas sign), external rotation of the hip (obturator sign), and shaking the patient's hips. Bowel sounds may be hypoactive or absent.

- Visceral pain should be distinguished from peritoneal pain because it indicates pathology of the abdominal contents without overt peritoneal irritation. This pain is often more poorly localized, the patient may writhe in pain, and there may be complete absence of focal tenderness to palpation.

Suggested Laboratory and Radiographic Studies in the Workup of Acute Abdominal Pain

Although not all of the following studies are indicated in each case of acute abdominal pain, the studies should be understood well so that they may be ordered appropriately.

- Pregnancy test should be performed for all female patients of reproductive age presenting with abdominal pain.
- CBC provides information about infection and anemia.
- Stool guaiac may diagnose occult gastrointestinal bleeding.
- UA may provide information about the presence of urinary tract infection or kidney stones.
- Liver function tests (aspartate aminotransferase [AST], alanine aminotransferase [ALT], bilirubin, alkaline phosphatase, and gamma glutamyl transferase [GGT]) may provide information about the presence of hepatic or biliary processes.
- Amylase and lipase may provide data about the presence of pancreatic disease.
- KUB (a plain abdominal radiograph of *k*idney, *u*reters, *b*ladder) may help identify bowel obstruction, perforation, or constipation. A KUB is indicated if significant vomiting is present (especially bilious vomiting) or if small or large bowel obstruction is suspected. It may also be used to screen for radiopaque kidney stones.
- Ultrasound is helpful in identifying gallstones, hydronephrosis, and sometimes appendicitis. However, not all cases of appendicitis are detected, especially in adults.
- CT scan is more expensive than ultrasound but may better visualize some organs. It may be ordered to help identify the cause of acute abdominal pain when an initial ultrasound yields equivocal results. Most cases of abdominal pain resulting from trauma warrant a CT scan. In addition, severe abdominal pain or significant abdominal pain with fever may warrant CT scanning.
- Intravenous pyelography (IVP) essentially is a KUB with IV contrast dye to image the upper urinary tract. It may help identify kidney stones.
- HIDA scan is a functional test of the gallbladder used for diagnosing acute cholecystitis and acalculous biliary disease. A HIDA scan often can be useful if a screening ultrasound is non-diagnostic in a patient suspected of having biliary disease.
- Upper GI with small bowel follow-through is a study in which the patient swallows oral contrast and fluoroscopic images are taken. This study may identify esophageal, gastric, and small bowel pathology.
- Endoscopy is the examination of the upper and/or lower GI tract using a fiberoptic scope. This study is invasive and requires specialty consultation. It may be helpful in diagnosing mucosal inflammation, polyps, and cancer. Endoscopy may be indicated in the workup of iron-deficiency anemia.

Classic Presentations of Common Diseases

Acute Appendicitis

Acute appendicitis commonly begins with anorexia, malaise, nausea/vomiting, and fever. Pain typically begins as diffuse periumbilical discomfort. Later, as the disease progresses, pain becomes localized to the right lower quadrant as peritoneal signs develop. UA is usually unremarkable. Elevation of the WBC is common. Radiographs may be normal, or may show a paucity of gas in the right lower quadrant or a calcification called an *appendolith*. CT scan usually reveals inflammation around the appendix. However, when acute appendicitis is suspected, CT scanning may be unnecessary as the patient may be taken to the operating for surgical exploration.

Urolithiasis

Urolithiasis, or kidney stones, typically presents with colicky unilateral flank pain with radiation to the ipsilateral groin or testicle as the stone encounters the ureteropelvic junction. Nausea and vomiting are common. Hematuria (gross or microscopic) is common. Fever and leukocytosis are absent unless a concomitant infection is present. As the stone passes distally, it encounters two additional areas of resistance, and pain often migrates. As the ureteral stone traverses the area of the iliac artery, lower abdominal pain develops. Later, when the stone encounters the ureterovesicular junction, suprapubic or groin pain may develop. The KUB may be normal unless the stone is radiopaque (e.g., calcium oxalate). A noncontrast abdominal CT is the diagnostic study of choice as it can reveal even radiolucent stones (e.g., uric acid). IVP may show ureteral obstruction or hydronephrosis. Renal ultrasound may also show hydronephrosis. Treatment for smaller stones (<4 mm) is generally symptomatic as these stones usually pass. Adequate analgesia can be provided with NSAIDs and narcotic analgesics (such as IV ketorolac with IV morphine or oral hydrocodone, oxycodone, hydromorphone). Hydration and straining the urine for stones is the mainstay of treatment. Larger stones or suspected infections require urologic consultation.

Cholelithiasis

Cholelithiasis (gallstones) typically presents as colicky right upper quadrant exacerbated by fatty meals. The pneumonic of the five F's often applies: the patient is "female, fat, forty, fair (Caucasian) and fertile." Pain may radiate to the right flank, back, or shoulders. Examination usually reveals tenderness in the right upper quadrant. With deeper palpation, as the patient inhales, there may be an abrupt halt in inspiration due to discomfort (Murphy's sign). Visceral pain is usual, but peritoneal signs may develop if there is significant inflammation or infection, as in cholecystitis and cholangitis.

Labs may include abnormal liver enzymes (AST, ALT, alkaline phosphatase, bilirubin), but this is highly variable. CBC and UA are normal in uncomplicated cases. Plain films typically are normal, particularly when infection is absent. A right upper quadrant ultrasound or CT scan may reveal stones in the gallbladder or common bile duct. MRI of the gallbladder and ducts magnetic resonance cholangiopancreatography (MRCP) may also be helpful. A HIDA scan may be helpful if the results of the previous scans are equivocal.

Medical treatment consists of analgesics, and antibiotics (such as cefotetan, ceftizoxime, and metronidazole) if infection is suspected. However, surgery is the definitive treatment in cholelithiasis. Stones may sometimes be removed via endoscopy.

Peptic Disease

Peptic disease usually presents as epigastric or substernal discomfort, which may be made worse (or better) with meals. Reflux of acid after meals or while supine suggests gastroesophageal reflux disease. Ulcers or gastritis/esophagitis and cancer may cause hematemesis (vomiting blood) or melena (black, tarry stools). Other potentially worrisome historical features include early meal satiety, unexplained anemia, weight loss, and dysphagia. The exam may be normal, or there may be epigastric tenderness to palpation.

Laboratory data such as CBC and UA typically is normal. If there is bleeding, a microcytic anemia, low serum iron, and positive stool guaiac are common. *H. pylori* antibodies or stool antigens may be positive. An upper GI series may reveal reflux or ulcers.

Treatment usually consists of an H2 blocker or a proton pump inhibitor. Antibiotics are often indicated if the patient has *H. pylori* infection to eradicate the presence of these bacteria. If malignancy is suspected, upper endoscopy is indicated.

Acute Diverticulitis

Diverticulitis is more common in patients over the age of 40. Signs and symptoms of infection very similar to appendicitis may be present. Typically, there is a predominance of left-sided symptoms as diverticular disease usually involves the descending colon and sigmoid colon. Fever, abdominal pain, and an elevated WBC may be present, but their frequency varies significantly. Initial visceral pain may progress to overt peritonitis.

CBC may reveal a normal or elevated WBC. Other labs are not necessary. As with appendicitis, perforation may be evident on plain films, showing subdiaphragmatic free air. CT scanning is helpful in identifying the location and extent of disease.

Treatment of diverticulitis includes antibiotics (in combinations such as ciprofloxacin with metronidazole or trimethoprim-sulfamethoxazole with metronidazole), bowel rest, and analgesics. Intravenous antibiotics are indicated if there is evidence of serious infection. Surgery or CT-guided drainage of abscess may be necessary if perforation occurs.

REFERENCES

American College of Emergency Physicians. Clinical policy: Critical issues for the initial evaluation and management of patients presenting with a chief complaint of nontraumatic acute abdominal pain. Ann Emerg Med 2000;36:4.

Carrico CW, Fenton LZ, Taylor GA, et al. Impact of sonography on the diagnosis and treatment of acute lower abdominal pain in children and young adults. Am J Roentgenol 1999;172:513–516.

Esses D, Birnbaum A, Bijur P, et al. Ability of CT to alter decision making in elderly patients with acute abdominal pain. Am J Emerg Med 2004;22(4); 270–272.

Ferozco LB, Raptopoulos V, Silen W. Acute diverticulitis. N Engl J Med 1998;38:1521–1526.

Graff LG, Robinson R. Abdominal pain and emergency department evaluation. Emerg Med Clin North Am 2001;19(1):123–136.

Kamin RA, Nowicki TA, Courtney DS, Powers RD. Pearls and pitfalls in the emergency department evaluation of abdominal pain. Emerg Med Clin North Am 2003;21(1):61–72.

Leung AK, Sigalet DL. Acute abdominal pain in children. Am Fam Physician 2003;7:2321–2326.

Trowbridge RL, Rutkowski NK, Shojania KG. Does this patient have acute cholecystitis? JAMA 2003;289:80–86.

Wagner JM, McKinney P, Carpenter JL. Does this patient have appendicitis? JAMA 1996;276:1589–1594.

Weyant MJ, Barie PS, Eachempati SR. Clinical role of noncontrast helical computed tomography in diagnosis of acute appendicitis. Am J Surg 2002; 183(1):97–99.

"My Arm Went Numb"

Examinee Prompt

You are seeing this 64-year-old patient in the emergency department for a chief complaint of "weakness." Please complete the following tasks:

- ❑ Obtain a focused history relevant to this patient's complaint
- ❑ Perform an appropriate physical examination

You will have 15 minutes to complete your visit with the patient. When you have all of the information that you need, you may leave the examination room. You do not need to explain your findings or your plan to the patient. Following your visit with the patient, please complete the following tasks:

- ❑ Write a "SOAP" (Subjective, Objective, Assessment and Plan) note, which should include your working diagnosis as well as a differential diagnosis to explain the patient's symptoms
- ❑ Outline your initial plan for the workup of this patient

Vital Signs

Temperature . . . . 99.1°F
Blood pressure . . . . 148/92 mm Hg
Pulse 84
Respiratory rate 16

Patient Prompt

Background: You are a 64-year-old patient who noticed weakness in your left arm while you were sitting and watching television.

Chief Complaint: Left arm weakness

History of the Present Illness: 64-year-old patient with an abrupt onset of left arm weakness while sitting and watching television. The weakness lasted 5 to 6 minutes and was not accompanied by any paresthesias. There was no headache, visual change, difficulty swallowing, difficulty with memory, difficulty speaking, or difficulty understanding speech. (Please provide this information to the examiner only if asked.) The arm simply felt heavy and difficult to control. There was no seizure activity or loss of consciousness. No fevers.

Past Medical History: Hyperlipidemia

Past Surgical History: Cholecystectomy age 42

Gynecologic History: G3P2 if female

Medications: Simvastatin 10 mg at night

Allergies: No known drug allergies

Family History:

- Father died of heart disease at age 84
- Mother alive and well at age 90
- No siblings
- No other significant family history

Social History:

- Retired from the police department
- Married with 3 grown children
- Lives with spouse
- One pack of cigarettes per day for 45 years
- Little physical activity

Review of Systems: Noncontributory except as noted in the history of the present illness

Additional Information:

- The physical examination is unremarkable in this case.
- If the examiner performs an eye examination, you may state that the funduscopic examination and pupillary reflexes are normal.
- If the examiner listens to the carotid arteries or heart, please state that the exam is unremarkable.
- Allow the examiner to perform a neurologic examination, but as the exam is performed, please state that each portion of the exam is normal.

Transient Ischemic Attack Scoresheet

Subjective

- ❑ Onset of symptoms
- ❑ Duration of symptoms
- ❑ Nature of symptoms
- ❑ Other associated neurologic symptoms (must ask for three, such as language difficulty, paresthesias, loss of balance, visual changes, etc.)
- ❑ Previous history of similar symptoms
- ❑ Headache
- ❑ Seizure activity
- ❑ Recent head trauma
- ❑ Past medical history
- ❑ Cigarette smoking
- ❑ Physical activity
- ❑ Medications
- ❑ Family history

Objective

- ❑ Funduscopic examination
- ❑ Auscultation of carotid arteries
- ❑ Cardiac examination
- ❑ Cranial nerve evaluation
- ❑ Limb strength
- ❑ Coordination (tandem gait or Romberg)
- ❑ Deep tendon reflexes
- ❑ Evaluation of sensation

Assessment

- ❑ The correct diagnosis of transient ischemic attack
- ❑ A differential diagnosis must be provided and should include at least three of the following (one point for each answer, 3 points maximum):
- ❑ Hypoglycemia or hyperglycemia
- ❑ Seizure disorder
- ❑ Hemorrhage (subarachnoid, subdural, etc.)
- ❑ Intracranial mass lesion
- ❑ Electrolyte disturbance
- ❑ Polycythemia
- ❑ Thrombocytopenia or thrombocythemia
- ❑ Complicated migraine
- ❑ Cervical radiculopathy

Plan (credit for up to five of the following items)

- ❑ Complete blood count (CBC)
- ❑ Chemistry panel (electrolytes, blood urea nitrogen, creatinine, glucose)
- ❑ Prothrombin time (PT), activated partial thromboplastin time (aPTT), international normalized ratio (INR)
- ❑ Head computed tomography (CT)
- ❑ Electrocardiogram (ECG)
- ❑ Carotid duplex ultrasonography
- ❑ Recommend smoking cessation

Total Score ____ / 30

Passing score for this station is 21 correct items.

Communication and Interpersonal Skills (CIS) Scoresheet

Please rate each of the following items on a scale from 1–10.
These items may be completed by either the standardized patient or another student.

Scoresheet 1

	Poor		Fair		Good		Very Good		Excellent	
Professional appearance	1	2	3	4	5	6	7	8	9	10
Introduces self and shakes hands	1	2	3	4	5	6	7	8	9	10
Nonverbal communication (eye contact, facial expressiveness, body language)	1	2	3	4	5	6	7	8	9	10
Communicates effectively (open-ended questions, avoids jargon)	1	2	3	4	5	6	7	8	9	10
Establishes rapport with patient (empathy, appears nonjudgmental)	1	2	3	4	5	6	7	8	9	10
Allows patient to speak without being interrupted	1	2	3	4	5	6	7	8	9	10
Listens and seems to understand patient's concerns	1	2	3	4	5	6	7	8	9	10
Overall professionalism	1	2	3	4	5	6	7	8	9	10

Total Score:

Passing score for CIS section is 56 points.

Spoken English Proficiency (SEP) Scoresheet

Please rate each of the following items on a scale from 1–10.
These items may be completed by either the standardized patient or another student.

Scoresheet 2

	Poor		Fair		Good		Very Good		Excellent	
Examiner is articulate and easily understood	1	2	3	4	5	6	7	8	9	10
Pronunciation (words pronounced correctly; accent does not hinder communication)	1	2	3	4	5	6	7	8	9	10
Word choice is appropriate	1	2	3	4	5	6	7	8	9	10
Ability to communicate without excessive listener effort required to understand questions or responses	1	2	3	4	5	6	7	8	9	10
Patient's ability to understand the examiner	1	2	3	4	5	6	7	8	9	10
Examiner's ability to understand the patient	1	2	3	4	5	6	7	8	9	10

Total Score:

Passing score for SEP section is 42 points.

Approach to the Patient with Suspected Transient Ischemic Attacks

Introduction

Transient ischemic attacks (TIAs) are defined as neurologic deficits caused by focal brain ischemia that resolve within 24 hours. Most TIAs last much less than 24 hours with most resolving within 1 hour. Recognizing TIA is of the utmost importance because it is a predictor of impending or future stroke. Patients who have had one or more TIAs have a 10-fold increase in the risk for subsequent stroke. As a result, TIA should be considered an ominous sign that merits early and aggressive evaluation and treatment.

Most TIAs are the result of an occlusion or partial occlusion of an artery supplying the brain. Most commonly, this vascular occlusion occurs as the result of a thromboembolic process due to atherosclerosis or embolism from a cardiac source. However, TIA may also result from hypercoagulable states, arteritis, and drugs of abuse such as cocaine.

TIAs often present as vague complaints that can be difficult to discern, particularly in patients who cannot provide accurate or thorough histories. The following list is a differential diagnosis of TIAs. Though a discussion of each of these topics is beyond the scope of this book, knowledge of this differential diagnosis is very important in clinical practice.

- Syncope
- Complicated migraine
- Multiple sclerosis
- Seizure
- Subarachnoid hemorrhage
- Hypoglycemia
- Neoplasm
- Vertigo
- Bell palsy
- Postictal paralysis (Todd paralysis)
- Neuromuscular disorders
- Functional disorders such as radiculopathy

Clinical Presentation

The clinical presentation of TIA depends upon whether the anterior or posterior circulation is affected. Interruption of blood flow in the anterior circulation results from embolic or thrombotic occlusion or stenosis of the carotid arteries. Ischemia in the areas of the brain served by the anterior circulation results in symptoms such as contralateral hemiparesis, contralateral sensory loss, disturbances in speech or language, ipsilateral monocular visual loss, and cognitive impairment.

TIAs occurring in the posterior circulation are more likely to result from thrombosis, but may result from rarer causes such as vertebral artery dissection. Ischemia in the areas of the brain served by the posterior circulation may result in vertigo, diplopia, dysphagia, homonomous hemianopia, ataxia, dysarthria, decreased level of consciousness, hemiparesis, and eye movement abnormalities.

The following list provides common clinical presentations of TIA. It should be remembered that TIA may present in atypical fashion, such as with inappropriate behavior or agitation.

- Unilateral or bilateral weakness affecting the face, arm, or leg
- Unilateral or bilateral sensory disturbance
- Unilateral or bilateral visual loss
- Double vision
- Difficulties with speech or language, such as slurring words, difficulty finding words, and difficulty with comprehension or pronunciation
- Difficulty swallowing
- Clumsiness or loss of balance
- Vestibular dysfunction
- Apathy or inappropriate behavior
- Somnolence
- Agitation
- Confusion or memory changes
- Inattention to the surrounding environment

Obtaining the History

The first step in evaluating a patient with symptoms that may be related to a TIA is to confirm the diagnosis. Much of this confirmation can be made with a thorough, focused history. The following items are important in evaluating the patient with suspected TIA.

- Patient age
- Onset of symptoms
- Duration of symptoms if symptoms have already resolved
- Past medical history and risk factors for TIA
  - Hypertension
  - Diabetes
  - Cardiac disease
  - Hyperlipidemia

  - Carotid artery stenosis
  - Tobacco use
  - Sickle cell anemia
  - Excessive alcohol use
  - Physical inactivity
  - Obesity
- Family history of stroke
- Medications
- Use of over-the-counter or illicit drugs
- History of recent head trauma (and associated head, neck, or jaw pain)
- History of migraine headaches (symptoms such as headache, nausea, and photophobia may suggest migraine rather than TIA)
- History of systemic clots or hypercoagulable states
- History of spontaneous abortion in a woman of childbearing age
- Recent fever

Physical Examination

The following physical examination items should be performed on all patients suspected of having TIA. If there are parts of the neurologic examination with which you are not comfortable, we recommend that you take the time to review a textbook of physical diagnosis to become more comfortable with the examination.

- Vital signs. The presence or absence of fever should be noted. Blood pressure should be obtained in both arms to rule out stenosis of the subclavian artery, which may manifest as significantly asymmetric blood pressures.
- Auscultation of the heart and carotid arteries.
- Detailed neurologic examination, including the following items:
  - Cognitive and language function
  - Cranial nerve function
  - Facial and limb strength
  - Sensory function
  - Deep tendon reflex symmetry
  - Coordination
  - Funduscopic examination and pupillary reflexes

Diagnostic Evaluation

Though there are no concrete guidelines for ancillary testing when TIA is suspected, there are current recommendations in the stroke literature. When TIA is suspected, the following tests should be performed in the initial evaluation:

- CBC to rule out polycythemia, thrombocytopenia, and thrombocytosis.
- PT, aPTT, and INR. These are helpful to know before antiplatelet or anticoagulation therapy is administered, as well as to help evaluate for some hypercoagulable states.
- Glucose level is used to rule out hypoglycemia or hyperglycemia as the cause of the patient's symptoms, as well as to diagnose occult diabetes.
- Electrolytes are measured because alterations in sodium levels may result in neurologic changes.
- Blood urea nitrogen (BUN) and creatinine are important because poor renal function may prohibit the use of contrast materials used in imaging studies.
- An erythrocyte sedimentation rate (ESR) is obtained to rule out vasculitis as the cause of symptoms.
- CT scan of the brain without contrast should be obtained to evaluate for subarachnoid hemorrhage, intracranial hemorrhage, subdural hematoma, and intracranial mass lesions.
- ECG with rhythm strip should be performed because atrial fibrillation and left ventricular hypertrophy are important risk factors for stroke and TIA. If the ECG is abnormal, echocardiography should be performed.
- Carotid duplex ultrasonography should be performed to exclude a flow-limiting lesion in the carotid arteries. Alternatively, vasculature may be evaluated by magnetic resonance angiography (MRA) with contrast or by CT angiography.

Management

After the initial evaluation of the patient with TIA, the first decision to make concerns the disposition of the patient. The disposition of a patient with suspected TIA requires great care because TIAs are a warning sign of an impending or future stroke. Although symptoms frequently resolve by the time the patient is evaluated by a physician, the serious nature of a TIA should not be discounted. It is the opinion of the authors, and much of the emergency medicine literature, that given the morbidity of TIA and stroke, few if any patients should be discharged home after the initial evaluation. There are no studies that help identify patients who can be safely evaluated on an outpatient basis. For these reasons, evaluation and management as an inpatient or in a disposition unit is recommended.

Treatment for patients with TIAs begins with risk factor modification. Modifiable risk factors for stroke and TIA include hypertension, cardiac disease (including atrial fibrillation), diabetes, cigarette smoking, hyperlipidemia, excessive alcohol use, physical inactivity, and stress.

For the patient admitted with TIA, blood pressure should not be treated aggressively immediately unless the systolic blood pressure is higher than 220 mm Hg or the diastolic blood pressure is above 120 mm Hg. This is because in patients with chronically elevated blood pressure, abrupt lowering of blood pressure could result in cerebral ischemia or worsening of an infarction. Exceptions include patients with acute myocardial infarction, hypertensive encephalopathy, renal failure, aortic dissection, or retinal hemorrhages.

Aspirin is the standard medical therapy used for prevention of ischemic stroke in patients who have had a TIA. The Food and Drug Administration and American Heart Association currently recommend the use of aspirin in doses of 50 mg/day to 325 mg/day for prevention of stroke and for TIA patients. Patients who suffer TIA while on daily aspirin therapy may be candidates for alternative antiplatelet agents or a combination of an alternative antiplatelet agent plus aspirin. These alternative agents include clopidogrel, ticlopidine, and extended-release dipyridamole with aspirin.

Treatment of Specific Cases

Atrial Fibrillation

Anticoagulation is recommended in patients with a TIA and atrial fibrillation who do not have contraindications to anticoagulation. Anticoagulation can be started using either intravenous unfractionated heparin or low-molecular-weight heparin while long-term therapy with warfarin sodium is being started. A target INR range of 2.0 to 3.0 is recommended. For the patient with atrial fibrillation who has contraindications to anticoagulation, antiplatelet therapy should be prescribed.

Carotid Stenosis

Atherosclerotic narrowing of the internal carotid artery is a common cause of TIA and stroke. Three major prospective randomized trials have evaluated the efficacy of carotid endarterectomy in symptomatic patients with high-grade carotid stenosis. The results of these trials show that symptomatic patients with 70% to 99% stenosis can expect a greater benefit from carotid endarterectomy than from medical therapy. Although new procedures such as vascular angioplasty and stenting have been developed, these procedures remain controversial in stroke prevention at this time.

Long-Term Management

For long-term reduction of stroke risk, the patient's modifiable risk factors should be addressed. After the immediate management of TIA and stroke, blood pressure should be reduced slowly over days to prevent worsening of ischemia. After discharge, the patient's blood pressure goal should be less than 140/90 mm Hg, or below 130/80 for the patient with diabetes or chronic renal disease.

The physician should make an attempt to encourage smoking cessation in all patients, but particularly in the patient who has had a TIA.

Patients with heart disease and atrial fibrillation in particular are at high risk for TIA or stroke. The patient's heart disease should be managed aggressively, and the patient with atrial fibrillation should be treated with anticoagulation therapy unless there are contraindications.

Diabetes increases stroke risk significantly. Though there is no conclusive evidence that tight glucose control results in a reduction of ischemic stroke, angiotensin-converting enzyme inhibitors may reduce cardiovascular and cerebrovascular events in patients with diabetes mellitus and one cardiac risk factor.

REFERENCES

Adams HP Jr, Adams RJ, Brott T, et al. Guidelines for the early management of patients with ischemic stroke: A scientific statement from the Stroke Council of the American Stroke Association. Stroke 2003;34:1056–1083.

Albers GW, Hart RG, Lutsep HL, Newell DW, Sacco RL. AHA scientific statement. Supplement to the guidelines for the management of transient ischemic attacks: A statement from the Ad Hoc Committee on Transient Ischemic Attacks, Stroke Council, American Heart Association. Stroke 1999;30: 2502–2511.

Atrial Fibrillation Investigators. Risk factors for stroke and efficacy of antithrombotic therapy in atrial fibrillation: Analysis of pooled data from five randomized controlled trials. Arch Intern Med 1994;154:1449–1457.

Beneficial effect of carotid endarterectomy in symptomatic patients with high-grade carotid stenosis. North American Symptomatic Carotid

Endarterectomy Trial Collaborators. N Engl J Med 1991;325:445–453.

Borg KT, Pancioli AM. Transient ischemic attacks: An emergency medicine approach. Emerg Med Clin North Am 2002;20:597–608.

Culebras A, Kase CS, Masdeu JC, et al. Practice guidelines for the use of imaging in transient ischemic attacks and acute stroke. A report of the Stroke Council, American Heart Association. Stroke 1997;28:1480–1497.

Effects of ramipril on cardiovascular and microvascular outcomes in people with diabetes mellitus; results of the HOPE study and MICRO-HOPE substudy. Heart Outcomes Prevention Evaluation Study Investigators [published correction appears in Lancet 2000;356:860]. Lancet 2000;355:253–259.

Elkins JS, Sidney S, Gress DR, et al. Electrocardiographic findings predict short-term cardiac morbidity after transient ischemic attack. Arch Neurol 2002;59: 1437–1441.

Feinberg W, Albers G, Barnett H, et al. Guidelines for the management of transient ischemic attacks. Stroke 1994;25(6):1320–1335.

Gerstein HC. Reduction of cardiovascular events and microvascular complications in diabetes with ACE inhibitor treatment: HOPE and MICRO-HOPE. Diabetes Metab Res Rev 2002;18(suppl 3):S82–S85.

Gorelick PB Sacco RL, Smith DB, et al. Prevention of a first stroke: A review of guidelines and a multidisciplinary consensus statement from the National Stroke Association. JAMA 1999;281:1112–1120.

Manktelow B, Gillies C, Potter JF. Interventions in the management of serum lipids for preventing stroke recurrence. Cochrane Database Syst Rev 2004;(1):CD002091.

Perkins GD. Mosby's Color Atlas and Text of Neurology. London, Mosby International, 1998, pp 113–118.

Reed DM, Resch JA, Hayaski T, MacLean C, Yano K. A prospective study of cerebral atherosclerosis. Stroke 1988;19:820–825.

Retinopathy and nephropathy in patients with type 1 diabetes four years after a trial of intensive therapy. The Diabetes Control and Complications Trial/Epidemiology of Diabetes Interventions and Complications Research Group [published correction appears in N Engl J Med 2000;342:1376]. N Engl J Med 2000;342:381–389.

Semplicini A, Maresca A, Boscolo G, et al. Hypertension in acute ischemic stroke: A compensatory mechanism or an additional damaging factor? Arch Intern Med 2003;163:211–216.

Solenski, NJ. Transient ischemic attacks: Part I. Diagnosis and evaluation. Am Fam Physician 2004;69:1665–1674.

Solenski NJ. Transient ischemic attacks: Part II. Treatment. Am Fam Physician 2004;69:1681–1688.

Straus SE, Majumdar SR, McAlister FA. New evidence for stroke prevention: Scientific review. JAMA 2002;288:1388–1395.

Index

Page numbers followed by f *indicate figures; those followed by* t *indicate tables.*

Additional Scoresheets

Communication and Interpersonal Skills (CIS) Scoresheet

Please rate each of the following items on a scale from 1–10.
These items may be completed by either the standardized patient or another student.

Scoresheet 1

	Poor		Fair		Good		Very Good		Excellent	
Professional appearance	1	2	3	4	5	6	7	8	9	10
Introduces self and shakes hands	1	2	3	4	5	6	7	8	9	10
Nonverbal communication (eye contact, facial expressiveness, body language)	1	2	3	4	5	6	7	8	9	10
Communicates effectively (open-ended questions, avoids jargon)	1	2	3	4	5	6	7	8	9	10
Establishes rapport with patient (empathy, appears nonjudgmental)	1	2	3	4	5	6	7	8	9	10
Allows patient to speak without being interrupted	1	2	3	4	5	6	7	8	9	10
Listens and seems to understand patient's concerns	1	2	3	4	5	6	7	8	9	10
Overall professionalism	1	2	3	4	5	6	7	8	9	10

Total Score:

Passing score for CIS section is 56 points.

Spoken English Proficiency (SEP) Scoresheet

Please rate each of the following items on a scale from 1–10.
These items may be completed by either the standardized patient or another student.

Scoresheet 2

	Poor		Fair		Good		Very Good		Excellent	
Examiner is articulate and easily understood	1	2	3	4	5	6	7	8	9	10
Pronunciation (words pronounced correctly; accent does not hinder communication)	1	2	3	4	5	6	7	8	9	10
Word choice is appropriate	1	2	3	4	5	6	7	8	9	10
Ability to communicate without excessive listener effort required to understand questions or responses	1	2	3	4	5	6	7	8	9	10
Patient's ability to understand the examiner	1	2	3	4	5	6	7	8	9	10
Examiner's ability to understand the patient	1	2	3	4	5	6	7	8	9	10

Total Score:

Passing score for SEP section is 42 points.

Communication and Interpersonal Skills (CIS) Scoresheet

Please rate each of the following items on a scale from 1–10.
These items may be completed by either the standardized patient or another student.

Scoresheet 1

	Poor		Fair		Good		Very Good		Excellent	
Professional appearance	1	2	3	4	5	6	7	8	9	10
Introduces self and shakes hands	1	2	3	4	5	6	7	8	9	10
Nonverbal communication (eye contact, facial expressiveness, body language)	1	2	3	4	5	6	7	8	9	10
Communicates effectively (open-ended questions, avoids jargon)	1	2	3	4	5	6	7	8	9	10
Establishes rapport with patient (empathy, appears nonjudgmental)	1	2	3	4	5	6	7	8	9	10
Allows patient to speak without being interrupted	1	2	3	4	5	6	7	8	9	10
Listens and seems to understand patient's concerns	1	2	3	4	5	6	7	8	9	10
Overall professionalism	1	2	3	4	5	6	7	8	9	10

Total Score:

Passing score for CIS section is 56 points.

Spoken English Proficiency (SEP) Scoresheet

Please rate each of the following items on a scale from 1–10.
These items may be completed by either the standardized patient or another student.

Scoresheet 2

	Poor		Fair		Good		Very Good		Excellent	
Examiner is articulate and easily understood	1	2	3	4	5	6	7	8	9	10
Pronunciation (words pronounced correctly; accent does not hinder communication)	1	2	3	4	5	6	7	8	9	10
Word choice is appropriate	1	2	3	4	5	6	7	8	9	10
Ability to communicate without excessive listener effort required to understand questions or responses	1	2	3	4	5	6	7	8	9	10
Patient's ability to understand the examiner	1	2	3	4	5	6	7	8	9	10
Examiner's ability to understand the patient	1	2	3	4	5	6	7	8	9	10

Total Score:

Passing score for SEP section is 42 points.

Communication and Interpersonal Skills (CIS) Scoresheet

Please rate each of the following items on a scale from 1–10.
These items may be completed by either the standardized patient or another student.

Scoresheet 1

	Poor		Fair		Good		Very Good		Excellent	
Professional appearance	1	2	3	4	5	6	7	8	9	10
Introduces self and shakes hands	1	2	3	4	5	6	7	8	9	10
Nonverbal communication (eye contact, facial expressiveness, body language)	1	2	3	4	5	6	7	8	9	10
Communicates effectively (open-ended questions, avoids jargon)	1	2	3	4	5	6	7	8	9	10
Establishes rapport with patient (empathy, appears nonjudgmental)	1	2	3	4	5	6	7	8	9	10
Allows patient to speak without being interrupted	1	2	3	4	5	6	7	8	9	10
Listens and seems to understand patient's concerns	1	2	3	4	5	6	7	8	9	10
Overall professionalism	1	2	3	4	5	6	7	8	9	10

Total Score:

Passing score for CIS section is 56 points.

Spoken English Proficiency (SEP) Scoresheet

Please rate each of the following items on a scale from 1–10.
These items may be completed by either the standardized patient or another student.

Scoresheet 2

	Poor		Fair		Good		Very Good		Excellent	
Examiner is articulate and easily understood	1	2	3	4	5	6	7	8	9	10
Pronunciation (words pronounced correctly; accent does not hinder communication)	1	2	3	4	5	6	7	8	9	10
Word choice is appropriate	1	2	3	4	5	6	7	8	9	10
Ability to communicate without excessive listener effort required to understand questions or responses	1	2	3	4	5	6	7	8	9	10
Patient's ability to understand the examiner	1	2	3	4	5	6	7	8	9	10
Examiner's ability to understand the patient	1	2	3	4	5	6	7	8	9	10

Total Score:

Passing score for SEP section is 42 points.

Communication and Interpersonal Skills (CIS) Scoresheet

Please rate each of the following items on a scale from 1–10.
These items may be completed by either the standardized patient or another student.

Scoresheet 1

	Poor		Fair		Good		Very Good		Excellent	
Professional appearance	1	2	3	4	5	6	7	8	9	10
Introduces self and shakes hands	1	2	3	4	5	6	7	8	9	10
Nonverbal communication (eye contact, facial expressiveness, body language)	1	2	3	4	5	6	7	8	9	10
Communicates effectively (open-ended questions, avoids jargon)	1	2	3	4	5	6	7	8	9	10
Establishes rapport with patient (empathy, appears nonjudgmental)	1	2	3	4	5	6	7	8	9	10
Allows patient to speak without being interrupted	1	2	3	4	5	6	7	8	9	10
Listens and seems to understand patient's concerns	1	2	3	4	5	6	7	8	9	10
Overall professionalism	1	2	3	4	5	6	7	8	9	10

Total Score:

Passing score for CIS section is 56 points.

Spoken English Proficiency (SEP) Scoresheet

Please rate each of the following items on a scale from 1–10.
These items may be completed by either the standardized patient or another student.

Scoresheet 2

	Poor		Fair		Good		Very Good		Excellent	
Examiner is articulate and easily understood	1	2	3	4	5	6	7	8	9	10
Pronunciation (words pronounced correctly; accent does not hinder communication)	1	2	3	4	5	6	7	8	9	10
Word choice is appropriate	1	2	3	4	5	6	7	8	9	10
Ability to communicate without excessive listener effort required to understand questions or responses	1	2	3	4	5	6	7	8	9	10
Patient's ability to understand the examiner	1	2	3	4	5	6	7	8	9	10
Examiner's ability to understand the patient	1	2	3	4	5	6	7	8	9	10

Total Score:

Passing score for SEP section is 42 points.

Communication and Interpersonal Skills (CIS) Scoresheet

Please rate each of the following items on a scale from 1–10.
These items may be completed by either the standardized patient or another student.

Scoresheet 1

	Poor		Fair		Good		Very Good		Excellent	
Professional appearance	1	2	3	4	5	6	7	8	9	10
Introduces self and shakes hands	1	2	3	4	5	6	7	8	9	10
Nonverbal communication (eye contact, facial expressiveness, body language)	1	2	3	4	5	6	7	8	9	10
Communicates effectively (open-ended questions, avoids jargon)	1	2	3	4	5	6	7	8	9	10
Establishes rapport with patient (empathy, appears nonjudgmental)	1	2	3	4	5	6	7	8	9	10
Allows patient to speak without being interrupted	1	2	3	4	5	6	7	8	9	10
Listens and seems to understand patient's concerns	1	2	3	4	5	6	7	8	9	10
Overall professionalism	1	2	3	4	5	6	7	8	9	10

Total Score:

Passing score for CIS section is 56 points.

Spoken English Proficiency (SEP) Scoresheet

Please rate each of the following items on a scale from 1–10.
These items may be completed by either the standardized patient or another student.

Scoresheet 2

	Poor		Fair		Good		Very Good		Excellent	
Examiner is articulate and easily understood	1	2	3	4	5	6	7	8	9	10
Pronunciation (words pronounced correctly; accent does not hinder communication)	1	2	3	4	5	6	7	8	9	10
Word choice is appropriate	1	2	3	4	5	6	7	8	9	10
Ability to communicate without excessive listener effort required to understand questions or responses	1	2	3	4	5	6	7	8	9	10
Patient's ability to understand the examiner	1	2	3	4	5	6	7	8	9	10
Examiner's ability to understand the patient	1	2	3	4	5	6	7	8	9	10

Total Score:

Passing score for SEP section is 42 points.